THE COMPLETE GUIDE TO

Soccer Fitness & Injury Prevention

THE COMPLETE GUIDE TO
Soccer Fitness &

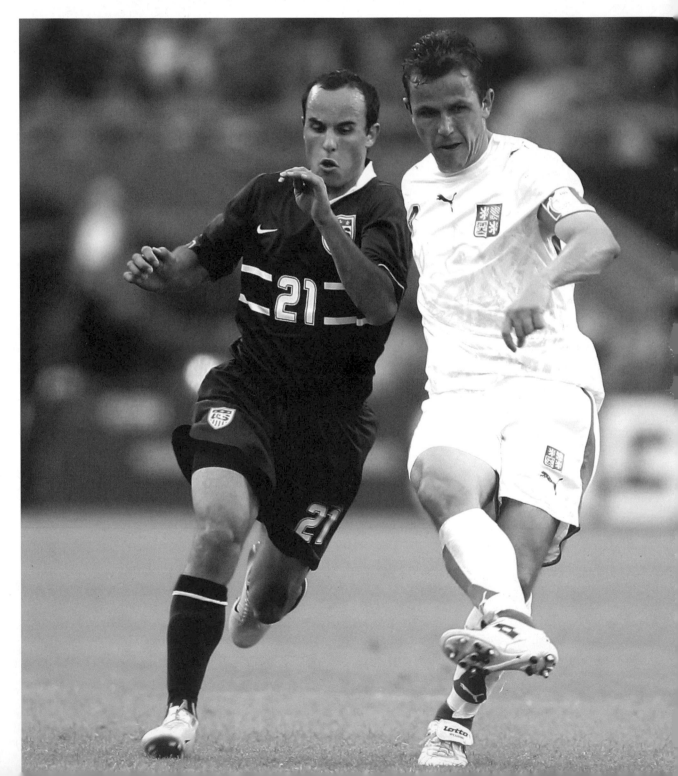

Injury Prevention

A Handbook for Players, Parents, and Coaches

DONALD T. KIRKENDALL

With clinical commentary by

WILLIAM E. GARRETT JR., M.D.

The University of North Carolina Press · Chapel Hill

© 2007 The University
of North Carolina Press
All rights reserved
Manufactured in the
United States of America
Designed and typeset
in The Serif and The Sans
by Eric M. Brooks

This book was published with
the assistance of the Blythe Family
Fund of the University of North
Carolina Press.

The paper in this book meets
the guidelines for permanence
and durability of the Committee
on Production Guidelines for
Book Longevity of the Council on
Library Resources.

Library of Congress
Cataloging-in-Publication Data
Kirkendall, Donald T.
The complete guide to soccer fitness and injury
prevention: a handbook for players, parents,
and coaches / Donald T. Kirkendall; with clinical
commentary by William E. Garrett Jr.
    p. cm.
Includes bibliographical references and index.
ISBN 978-0-8078-3182-3 (cloth: acid-free paper)
ISBN 978-0-8078-5857-8 (pbk.: acid-free paper)
1. Soccer injuries. I. Garrett, William E. II. Title.
RC1220.S57K57   2007
617.1'027—dc22   2007019052

cloth   11 10 09 08 07   5 4 3 2 1
paper   11 10 09 08 07   5 4 3 2 1

CONTENTS

In the mid-1980s I managed to get myself on the program of the National Soccer Coaches Association of America (NSCAA) to talk about nutrition and soccer. At that meeting I wandered into a scheduled, yet casual, meeting of NSCAA's *Soccer Journal* and asked the editor, Tim Schum of the State University of New York at Binghamton, if the journal would be interested in some sports science articles. Tim said yes, and since then I've been writing about sports science topics as applied to soccer for coaches, players, and parents in various outlets like the *Soccer Journal, Southern Soccer Scene*, Active.com, the U.S. Soccer Federation website, and some FIFA (Fédération Internationale de Football Association) sources.

I have spent the last 10 years working for and with Dr. William E. Garrett Jr., and we have collaborated on many sports medicine topics. As is the case with most professionals in sports medicine, we have a sport of particular interest, and our joint interest in soccer is probably what helped draw us together. Dr. Garrett has the experience in the medical aspects of soccer, and my expertise is in the coaching and fitness side of the sport. When the concept of the book was in development, it was obvious that both of us should prepare the content. We decided that I should author the text, and Dr. Garrett would make comments based on his experiences as a team physician for high school, university, and U.S. Soccer national teams.

The goal in preparing this book is to help parents, coaches, and players be better prepared for the physical aspects of the game. My experience comes as much from the exercise sciences and the clinic as from my days playing on the field, coaching on the sideline, and rehabbing in the training room. The text here expands on pieces I have written for various outlets. It is my hope that players will approach the game with more awareness of the role of fitness in performance and injury prevention, which will make the game more fun to play and more enjoyable to watch.

This book, to steal FIFA's motto, is "for the good of the game."

Many friends, colleagues, and mentors have helped guide and accompany me on this journey deep into soccer. My mom and dad gave me every opportunity to feed my soccer jones, but they only got to see me play once, which I regret to this day.

Many people had an impact on my interest in soccer and sports science, even though they may not realize it. I stand on the shoulders of many giants:

- In the exercise sciences, Fritz Hagerman, who was as skilled with a pat on the back as he was with a foot in the backside; Dave Costill; Duane Eddy; Bud Getchell; Reggie Edgerton; the late Ed Fox; Bob Bartels; Carl Foster; the late Ed Burke; Ron Maughan; Fred Mueller; Bing Yu; Kevin Guskiewicz; Ruben Echemendia; Anders Ericsson; Tom Reilly; Jens Bangsbo (and his colleagues Magni Mohr and Peter Krustrup); and Turibio Barros are at the top of the list. Add to that list all the folks I worked with at the K-Lab at Duke University, especially Patty Marchak and Tony Seaber, and at the Sports Medicine Research Lab and the Center for Human Movement Science at the University of North Carolina at Chapel Hill.
- In soccer, the late Andy Smiles and Ed Roberts—Ohio University teammates—helped me become a starter and showed me what real passion for the game meant. Thanks also to the rest of the Ohio University team, who demanded total immersion in the game, as well as the players I coached at Ball State.
- Coaching friends whose influence can be seen herein include Anson Dorrance (and his staff, Bill Pallindino, Chris Ducar, Tom Sander, and Greg Gatz), Elmar Bolowich, John Ellinger, Jerre McManama, Bill Barfield, Ralph Lundy, Thomas Rongren, the late Clive Charles, Tony DiCicco, April Heinrichs, Tracey Leone, Steve Sampson, Timo Liekoski, Jay Hoffman, Bruce Arena, Pierre Barrieu, Lee Horton, Tim Schum, Ray Alley, Vern Gambetta, and the staff of the North Carolina Youth Soccer Association. The teaching staff at the U.S. Soccer coaching school, which I attended in 1975, really showed me what was necessary and how little I knew about coaching—the late

Walt Chyzowich, Bill Muse, Nick Zlater, Lenny Lucencko, and Joe Machnick.

• At the U.S. Soccer Federation, many of the administrators have been more than accommodating with my queries and access to the national teams program, but none more than Hughie O'Malley.

• I am also grateful to Jirí Dvorák, director of F-MARC (FIFA Medical Assessment and Research Centre), the research arm of FIFA, for the opportunity to work in some small way "for the good of the game" at the international level.

• In sports medicine, many physicians have influenced what is said here. These include John Bergfeld, Gary Weiker, Jack Andrish, and John Lombardo, all of the Cleveland Clinic, as well as Roald Bahr, Lars Petersen, John Feagin, and, most important, the two lead physicians for U.S. Soccer: Bert Mandelbaum, who helped open the door to F-MARC, and Bill Garrett Jr., who created the opportunity to work with U.S. Soccer and FIFA and taught me more about injuries than he'll ever realize.

Introduction

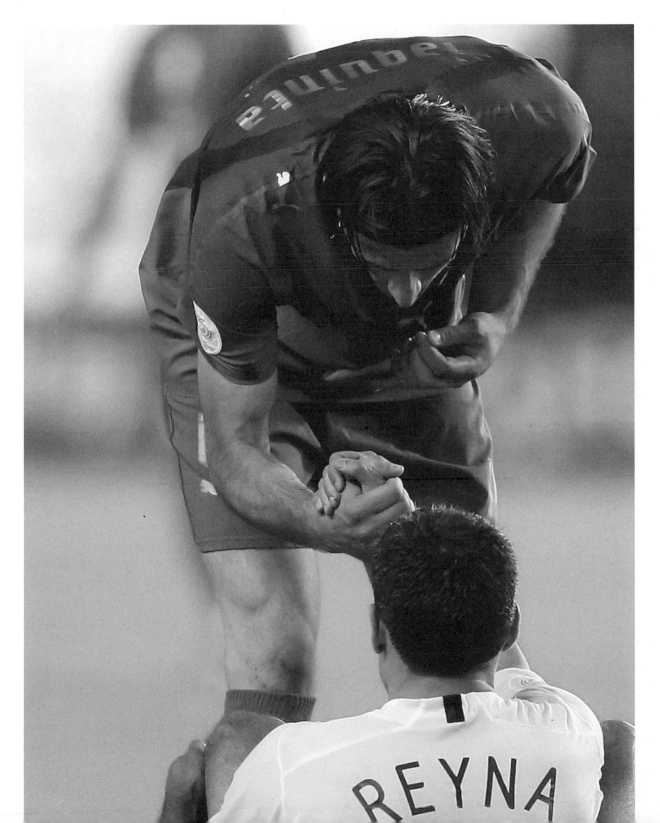

Soccer has been called "the beautiful game," as well as "the simplest game." We can all identify with the description "the beautiful game": quality soccer is beautiful. Most fans of the sport can recall specific matches or plays that bear out their definition of beauty.

Most fans have more difficulty in describing just what makes soccer "the simplest game." They may begin by pointing out that there are few rules. The laws of the game number only seventeen, and most of these define game length, field size, ball dimensions, player uniforms, referee duties, and the like; only two laws (#11—offsides and #12—fouls and misconduct) describe fouls and infractions. Other people may also say something about the most basic athletic confrontation—one versus one—and the way the game leads to those situations. Most fans overlook basic information about the game they all love, however. How many possessions does a team get during a game? And how many players actually touch the ball during a possession? What is the best way to get a shot on goal? We all find dribbling beautiful, but when a team gets a shot or a score, was dribbling involved? The overarching question is whether we really know what all is going on during a match.

It is very difficult to train for a game if you don't know the game. You wouldn't train a soccer player like a basketball player, nor would you train a basketball player like a middle-distance runner. To understand training and to prevent injuries, you need to understand the nature of the game. It would help if you knew, for example, how far and fast a player runs. This kind of information can only come from a continuing study of actual games.

One of the first amateur teams I played for was supported by a German American social club, and we got plenty of help from guys from the "old country" that was really quite useful as we prepared for matches. I learned back then that knowing what *was* done was as important as finding out what *is* done. So, many new insights can come from observations made many years ago:

> Football is a simple game. The hard part is making it look simple.
> (Ron Greenwood, England manager, 1978)

> It took me 16 years to realize this is a passing, not a dribbling game.
> (Jimmy Hill, Fulham player, 1970s)

A player receiving a pass has two feet, but only one head.
(Willie Read, Scotland manager, 1959)

Make it simple, make it accurate, make it quick.
(Arthur Rowe, *Encyclopedia of Association Football*, 1960)

I like Willie Read's comment; it sounds like the old Vince Lombardi quip about passing the football: he said that only three things come from a pass, and two of them are bad. But Read's comment is wise: keep the ball on the ground. Paul Gardner, the *Soccer America* columnist, has come up with something similar as one of his guides to quality soccer—the more time the ball spends in the air, the lower the quality of play.

Although one of the first things we teach children in soccer is dribbling, it really looks like soccer is a passing, not a dribbling, game. Keep the ball on the ground, and be both accurate and quick with the ball. In the 1960s a British mathematician, the late wing commander Charles Reep, watched hundreds of soccer games at all levels of play and noted that around 90% of all team possessions began and ended with three or fewer completed passes. In the mid-1970s Tom Reilly and his colleagues from Liverpool John Moores University in England studied every match activity of Everton FC during a professional season. They were the first to quantify the total distance run in a game—over 8,500 meters—and they found that a single player performed over 800 discrete activities each game (this is where the guys from the "old country" were off a bit: they said a player ran 10 miles). This works out to a change of speed or direction every 5–6 seconds. These findings provided valuable information on how specific training might be directed.

Reilly also showed that the average player was in control of the ball for only 90 seconds in the whole game and for a total of fewer than 200 meters. He put numbers to the obvious: a player spends far more time without the ball. This is why coaches tell their players that they should *always* be thinking of how to get the ball, whether they are on offense or defense:

You play 19/20 of the game without the ball ... when you
do your real thinking ... when you do your real playing.
(Arthur Rowe, 1960)

We improved … "kick and run" to "pass accurately and run into a good position." (Ferenc Puskas, Hungarian national team, 1953)

The good player keeps playing even without the ball … placing himself so that when the ball comes to him he is able to make good use of it. (Ferenc Puskas, 1953)

Speaking of history, if you don't know anything about the Hungarian national team of the mid-1950s, you should. (You may have heard about its 6-3 demolition of England at Wembley in 1953, but the rematch the next year in Hungary was even more lopsided at 7-1.) The game we love today reflects much of how the Hungarians changed the way the game was played.

I've summarized Reilly's original work in table 1.1. What we see is that about two-thirds of the men's game in the English professional league of the mid-1970s was played at the aerobic lower intensities of a walk or a jog, and the remaining third was at the higher intensities of a cruise ("running with manifest purpose and effort") and sprinting. In addition, sprint distances were shown to rarely exceed 40 meters. In the modern game the total running distance has now increased to 10–12 kilometers for professional men and 8–9 kilometers for women, with some Women's United Soccer Association (WUSA) players covering 10 kilometers like the men. Think about that: Women today cover the distances that professional men covered in the 1970s. What should you take from this? Concentrate on endurance, don't neglect sprint training, but keep the sprint distances to 40–50 meters and less. The hard part is how you train for endurance within the structure of the game.

AT SOME POINT, YOU HAVE TO GET THE BALL FROM THE OPPONENTS

I don't know about you, but I get a little tired of hearing whether a National Football League team plays the West Coast Offense, or a three-man versus four-man front, or zone or man defense. In contrast, the discussion among soccer coaches, fans, and television commentators revolves around the system a team plays—that is, how the players are arranged. What is the better system? 4-4-2? 4-3-3? 3-4-3? 4-5-1? Man marking or zone coverage? Possession or counterattacking? What about the old 2-3-5 or the "W" or "M" formation? If you have

I'm not here to play fitba', I'm here to see you don't play fitba'. (Attributed to an R. S. McColl, Glasgow Rangers center half, 1890s)

It is much easier to destroy than it is to create. (Ubiquitous coaching advice)

TABLE I.1

Movement Patterns in Soccer

Activity	% Total Distance	% Movement
Walking	25	36
Jogging	37	28
Cruising	21	14
Sprinting	11	7
Backing up	6	14

Source: T. Reilly and V. Thomas, "A Motion Analysis of Work Rate in Different Positional Roles in Professional Football Match Play," *Journal of Human Movement Studies* 2 (1976): 87–97.

Note: 850–1,000 discrete activities were identified over a total distance of 10 kilometers.

not already thought about it, most of these formations are defensive formations—what kind of barrier is presented to the opponents and then how to attack from it. Coaching gurus probably have much more to say on that. Currently, the 4-4-2 changes to sort of a 2-4-4 when on offense, with the wing midfielders moving up to become wing forwards and with wing defenders moving up a line, then both returning when on defense. In the 1960s the late Woody Hayes, legendary football coach of Ohio State University, wrote a book entitled *You Win with People*. What Hayes was saying is that one should find the best players first and then design the system around their abilities. The best coaches adapt the playing style of their team to the abilities of their players, not vice versa. At the 1996 Olympics, Tony DiCicco, coach of the gold medal U.S. women's team, used man marking and a sweeper. At the 1999 Women's World Cup, with some new players, he changed to zonal marking for a flat back four defense. He didn't change just because everybody else was changing. His mix of players had changed. (There still are successful teams playing with a traditional sweeper—the 2004 European champion Greece, for example; there's nothing wrong with that; what goes around comes around.)

There are almost as many systems as there are ways to divide ten players into three or four lines. A lifelong friend of mine, Ralph Lundy, now at the College of Charleston, used to be at Erskine College in South Carolina. For a period of time, he had probably one of the very best players in the National Association of Intercollegiate Athletics (NAIA). When asked what system Erskine was playing, Ralph said a box-and-

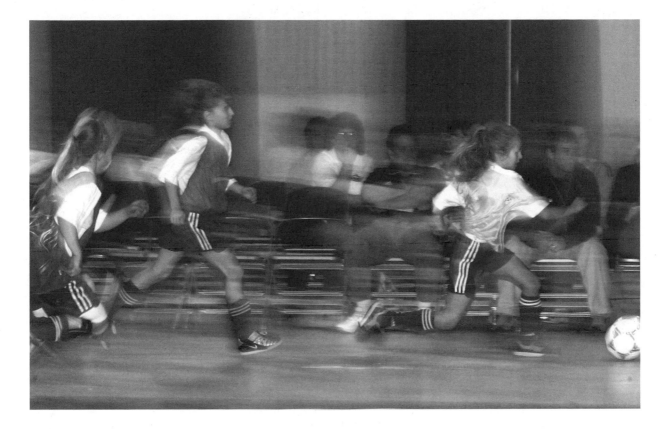

one. Wait a minute, you might be thinking, that's basketball, Ralph. Not for him. He lined up his team in a 3-3-3 formation and allowed his superstar to do anything he wanted. His players had to execute the system the best way possible, offensively and defensively. Develop the system to fit the players, not the players to fit the system.

Team defense eventually comes down to individual or small-group defensive tactics. While data regarding offensive tactics are kept, little is reported on individual defensive skills. In table 1.2 I list the main ways the ball changed possession during six randomly selected games from the 1998 France World Cup. The primary method of obtaining possession was following a mistake by the opposition: the opponent executed a trap, dribble, or pass poorly. This could have been the result of either pressure by the defending team or a simple skill error. Change of possession by a foul, tackle, ball going out of play, or a shot was fairly even. Thus, it looks like change of possession is more a function of small-group tactics to force an error, leading to an easily controlled free ball.

Speed is a fitness factor that may improve only slightly with training, but it is likely to be the factor that decides the outcome of a match. Many coaches look for the fast, skilled player, knowing they can improve the other aspects of fitness. (Photograph by Tony Quinn; SoccerStock.com)

TABLE I.2

Losing Possession of the Ball

	% of Lost Possessions
Bad pass	39
Foul	14
Tackle	13
Out of play	13
Shot	12

Source: Donald T. Kirkendall, "The Nature of the Game," in *International Football Sports Medicine: Caring for the Soccer Athlete Worldwide*, ed. Jirí Dvorák and Donald T. Kirkendall (Rosemont, Ill.: American Orthopaedic Society for Sports Medicine, 2005).

Note: Data come from a review of Men's and Women's World Cup matches.

ON SCORING A GOAL

Soccer lovers frequently describe their game as 90 minutes of constant action. Sorry, but the ball is actually in play for around 60 to 70 minutes. The rest of the time the ball is out of play ("out of touch," if you want to speak the way the Europeans do). Such situations include times when the ball is being moved to the proper spot following a foul, players are waiting for the wall to be properly set, or the ball is being retrieved after an off-target shot or set up for a penalty kick (what the English call a "spot" kick). An example from the women's world championship of 1991 is shown in figure I.1. Each stoppage might seem fairly brief, but all these seconds add up over the course of a game. The weather can also affect the amount of time the ball is in play. Excessive heat and high altitude will slow down a game, as players are not as eager to retrieve the ball for the restart of play. At the 1986 World Cup in Mexico, during a game played in group play at altitude on an unusually hot day, the ball was only in play for 45 minutes.

A few years ago, in 1994, a summary of goals scored in the Scottish Football League according to time was published in the *International Review for the Sociology of Sport*. The number of goals tended to increase as the game progressed, most likely due to player fatigue. A similar trend can be seen in goals over a season of play in U.S. Major League Soccer. The trend from the 1999 Women's World Cup is a little different, where goals were a little more evenly spread out over the game (figure I.2).

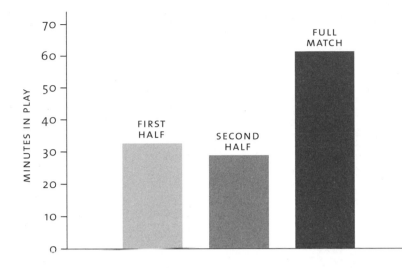

FIGURE I.1

Time Ball Was in Play,
1991 Women's World Cup

There are plenty of characteristics of the game that seem to have withstood the test of time. For example, the typical ratio of shots to goals is 10 to 1, and the average number of goals per game is between 1.5 and 2, depending on the setting. A devotee of Wing Commander Reep, Neil Lanham, reports that there are about 240 changes of possession in a game. Figuring in goals scored, he shows that there is one goal in about 180 possessions. Who wins? About 85% of the time, the team that scores first wins the game. Here is something to watch for in future world championships. In the men's World Cup, teams that lose the opening game of group play rarely advance to the elimination round. Another apparent correlation, sort of an "urban legend" about the World Cup, is that the team that scores first in the final loses the final. This isn't true for every final match, but it occurs often enough that commentators will bring it up when the first goal is scored. (France scored first and eventually lost to Italy in 2006.)

In his studies Reep followed recreational and professional soccer play and focused on the number of passes per possession for all possessions. If one focuses only on shooting and scoring possessions, the patterns still parallel Reep's observations. According to statistics gathered from multiple games in the late 1990s and early 2000s, when the U.S. women's national team obtained possession in the offensive third of the field, a shooting possession averaged two players and one pass. In this strategy, a team member obtains possession and passes

FIGURE I.2

When Are Goals Scored?

Sources: Scottish Football League data from Richard Guilianotti, "Scoring Away from Home: A Statistical Study of Scotland Football Fans at International Matches in Romania and Sweden," *International Review for the Sociology of Sport* 29, no. 2 (1994): 171–99; Major League Soccer data for the 2005 season from <MLSnet.com>.

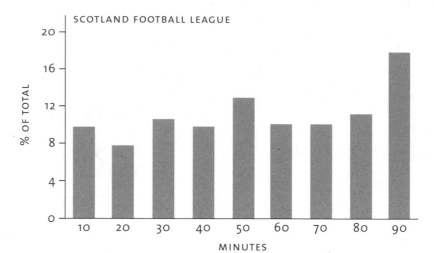

SCOTLAND FOOTBALL LEAGUE

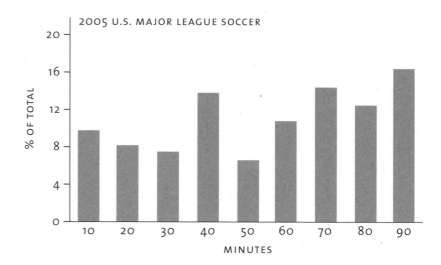

2005 U.S. MAJOR LEAGUE SOCCER

to the most dangerous player, who then shoots. When possession began in the middle third of the field, three players and two passes led to a shot. When possession was obtained in the defensive third, six players and five passes led to a shot. At a "lower" level (U.S. collegiate women), these numbers were similar for the possessions that began in the offensive and middle thirds of the field, but the collegiate players were more direct to the shot from the defensive third (mostly from a "clear"). High school females tend to play a more direct pattern, probably due to lower skill level (table 1.3).

Once shots are taken, a probability of scoring can be estimated (figure 1.3). Scoring probability in the goal box and the penalty area is

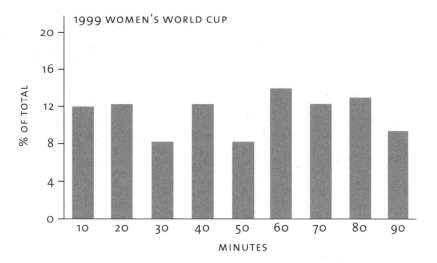

1999 WOMEN'S WORLD CUP

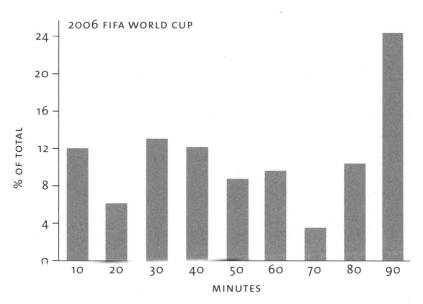

2006 FIFA WORLD CUP

Field Position	National Team	College	High School
Defensive third	4.9	3.2	1
Middle third	2.4	1.9	1.4
Offensive third	1.1	1.2	.67

TABLE 1.3

Number of Passes to a Shot in Women's Soccer by Ability Level and Field Position

Source: Donald T. Kirkendall, "The Nature of the Game," in *International Football Sports Medicine: Caring for the Soccer Athlete Worldwide*, ed. Jirí Dvorák and Donald T. Kirkendall (Rosemont, Ill.: American Orthopaedic Society for Sports Medicine, 2005).

FIGURE 1.3

Probability of Scoring by Ability
Level and Shooting Location
Source: Adapted from Donald T.
Kirkendall, "The Nature of the Game," in
*International Football Sports Medicine:
Caring for the Soccer Athlete Worldwide*,
ed. Jirí Dvorák and Donald T. Kirkendall
(Rosemont, Ill.: American Orthopaedic
Society for Sports Medicine, 2005).

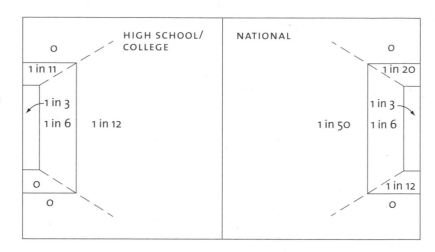

similar for female players across experience levels, but the chance of scoring from longer range is poor for the national team players, which suggests that they are facing better goalkeepers, not that the younger players are better long-range shooters.

Comparing Goals from the Men's and Women's World Cup

Let me try to compare apples and apples by analyzing the men's and women's game using results from similar tournaments, the 1998 and 1999 World Cups, respectively, from the knock-out round through the final.

The first comparison looks at when during a match goals were scored (figure 1.4). The men scored both early and late in the second half, whereas the women scored most of their goals at the opening of each half. This might suggest a fundamental difference in how men and women approach their game. Men might "probe" for weaknesses and exploit what they learn from the first half early in the second half and then again at the end of the game as players tire. The better women's teams try to put their opponent on their heels early in the match, forcing them to stretch their play and become more open for counterattacks. At the world level, there is a wider spread of abilities between the women's teams than between the men's teams.

The number of players and passes per shooting possession for women is similar to that found by Charles Reep (figure 1.5). The men, however, were at the low end of numbers of players and passes per

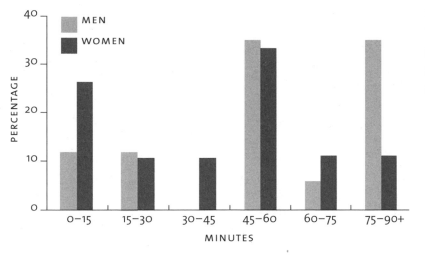

FIGURE I.4

Time of Goal by Sex

Source: Based on data collected by
the author, 1998 Men's World Cup and
1999 Women's World Cup.

possession. In figure I.6 the data for completed passes by men and women in the 1998 and 1999 World Cup tournaments are superimposed with Reep's work to show similarities and differences.

From all this data, we can generate scoring probabilities (figure I.7). The probability of scoring in the penalty area was similar for men and women, but shooting close in and at long range favored the women. This discrepancy could indicate that male goalkeepers are more commanding of the area immediately in front of the goal and are better at handling long-range shots. Women's coaches like Tony DiCicco and April Heinrichs have spoken about this difference in goalkeeping abilities, as well as the need for goalkeepers with better foot skills.

Overall, combining the men's and women's data, the shot to goal ratio was 9.25 to 1. Men scored 65% of their goals from free play, and women scored 79% of their goals from free play. Shooting drills in training should reflect what goes on in the game: 85% of the shots in the goal box were one-touch; 70% in the penalty area were one-touch, while only 45% of long-range shots were one-touch. Outside the penalty area, shots were set up with some dribbling. The women began 79% of their scoring possessions in the offensive third of the field, while the men began their scoring possessions equally in the offensive and middle thirds of the field (41% each). Overall, a typical scoring play involved four players and three passes, usually began in the offensive third (women) or offensive two-thirds (men), and rarely involved square or back passing. Ever wonder why so many people

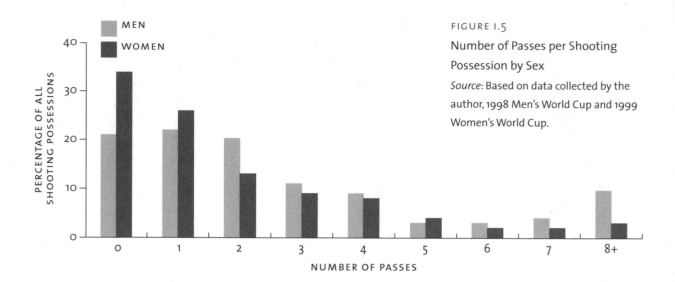

FIGURE 1.5

Number of Passes per Shooting Possession by Sex

Source: Based on data collected by the author, 1998 Men's World Cup and 1999 Women's World Cup.

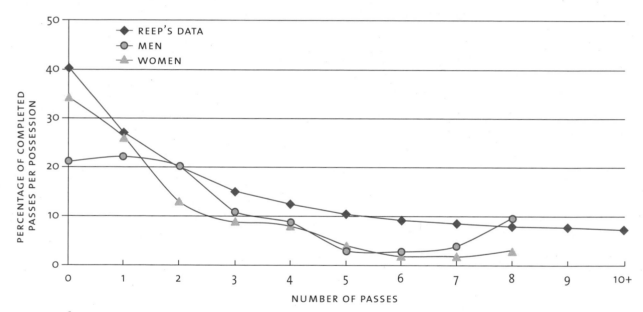

FIGURE 1.6

Proportion of Completed Passes

Sources: Based on data in C. Reep and B. Benjamin, "Skill and Chance in Association Football," *Journal of the Royal Statistical Society*, ser. A, 131, no. 4 (1968): 581–85, and men's and women's data collected by the author, 1998 Men's World Cup and 1999 Women's World Cup.

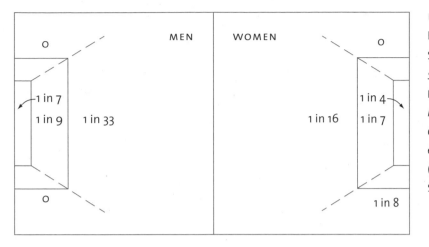

FIGURE I.7

Probability of Scoring by
Sex and Shooting Location
Source: Adapted from Donald T.
Kirkendall, "The Nature of the Game," in
*International Football Sports Medicine:
Caring for the Soccer Athlete Worldwide*,
ed. Jirí Dvorák and Donald T. Kirkendall
(Rosemont, Ill.: American Orthopaedic
Society for Sports Medicine, 2005).

recommend 4v4 as an ideal training game? A soccer match is less an 11v11 game and more a series of smaller 4v4 games. The 4v4 game not only gives each player more ball contacts and keeps all players more involved in play, but it also mimics the true nature of soccer. (In the 2006 World Cup, Argentina scored from a twenty-five pass combination. But how often is that going to happen?)

POSSESSION OR MISTAKES?

Watch soccer very closely, and you will see that most possessions begin with an error, followed by a quick decision for a penetrating dribble or pass that places the defensive team at a numerical disadvantage. Brazil plays "the beautiful game"—a wonderful display of multiple passes and brilliant dribbling—don't they? Yet even Brazil rarely scores from possessions of ten to twelve passes. They are no different from anyone else. When the opportunity to attack the goal occurs, all good teams react the same way, by attacking rapidly with numbers. The challenge of coaching is teaching players to recognize the opportunity when it arises and to make the best run to take advantage of it:

> A team *must* be able to play both possession and direct. Possession to force a team to chase . . . then recognize the opportunity to play direct. (Tony DiCicco, coach of the U.S. women's national team, 1999 Women's World Cup champions)

Possession and patience are myths. . . . Goals come from mistakes, not possession. (Graham Taylor, Watford manager, 1982)

Good teams make you pay for your mistakes. Great teams make you pay for your only mistake. (Alexi Lalas, on Italy's 1-0 defeat of the United States, *USA Today*, 14 February 2002)

I've presented a lot of numbers and concepts thus far, but the bottom line is that to improve, you have to learn the game and play the game as it is really played.

Perhaps, unfortunately, youth sports today have taken on a role that was barely discussed a generation ago. For many, athletic excellence is a ticket to a "free" college education. Major League Soccer's signing in 2004 of then 14-year-old Freddy Adu will make some parents think of youth soccer as a path to a professional contract, but Freddy is hardly the first American to go straight from high school to the pros. Others include Landon Donovan, DaMarcus Beasley, Bobby Convey, Santino Quaranta, and a number of others, many of whom came through the U.S. Soccer Federation's under-17 residential program in Bradenton, Florida.

Yet the odds work against either occurrence. There are around 200 National Collegiate Athletic Association (NCAA) Division I universities with men's soccer teams. If one assumes each school can offer the full complement of eleven scholarships (a suspect assumption), that would mean there is the dollar equivalent of 2,200 full scholarships. (Most scholarship money is split among multiple players, however, meaning there are very, very few of the classic "full rides" awarded.) The coach who has planned well will only have one-quarter of the dollars to award each year (to spread the money out over 4 years), meaning there are around 440 full scholarships (or the equivalent) available each year, and the competition for those limited dollars is intense indeed.

The overall goal of the coach is to teach the game to his or her players and develop players to grow in the game. Some parents have put another responsibility on the coach: if a player does not win a scholarship, it must be someone's fault. Players now compete in an inordinate number of games and competitions each year in an often ill-fated attempt at development and visibility. Talking about reducing the number of games played, however, is like talking about the weather: lots of talk but not much action.

Many people today say players are competing way too much and practicing too little. People experienced in sports know that development in a particular sport is related first and foremost to practice, not competition. When players compete without enough practice, they are cautious in trying new techniques and strategies to the point of even playing slower and more conservatively during tournaments. Skills are not honed this way. Union of European Football Associations (UEFA) research has shown that an increased match density prior to the 2002 World Cup led players to poorer performance and a higher injury rate, as compared with players with a lower match density. I've even heard of some youth playing upward of 140 games in a calendar year. When do they train?

We've all heard the great names, many recognizable by one name: Pelé, Johann, Diego, The Kaiser, Mia, Beckham, Ronaldo, and many more. Ever wondered just what it takes to become a superior athlete? We give genetics credit for everything these days, so why not athletic prowess? Maybe genetics play a role in basketball, where height is a plus—you can't "train" height. Maybe the extreme mass of football players has a genetic link, but they also do a lot of weight training to increase muscle mass (and eat a lot, too). What about soccer? A selling point of soccer is that it is a game that requires no particular genetic gifts to be successful. You might gawk at Shaquille O'Neal at 7 feet and 300 pounds of chiseled muscle, but most of the soccer elite wouldn't turn your head if you saw them at the mall. Pelé? He's 5 feet, 9 inches tall. U.S. forward Landon Donovan could pass for a video store clerk. You might see Cat (Reddick) Whitehill, a defensive starter on the U.S. women's national team, in the food court, and your friend would say there is no way she is a world-class soccer player. However, there is something different about these individuals that led to their success in the game. Practice. Deliberate practice.

Anson Dorrance frequently points out that he knew Mia Hamm was a great player when he first saw her, but he didn't realize her commitment until he drove by the field in February, the collegiate off-season, and saw her bent over from exhaustion because she had been training—alone. I watched the 1996 women's Olympic team doing a killer training workout, the kind that most of us would never, ever contemplate. Tony DiCicco was urging them on with "Faster, *faster*, this is why we're the best in the world." Lauren Gregg, Tony's longtime assistant, was coaching an under-20 women's national team when they were being tested for their fitness—tests of physical, as well as mental, dedication that demand work beyond the pain of fatigue. All the while she was driving them with "Come on, it's what we do when no one is watching that makes us champions."

You might say that these are just old coaching slogans to motivate players. There is only so much that a coach can do, however. The player who really wants to be exceptional has a responsibility to keep working when no one is watching, when the pain of fatigue and the boredom of repetition make the body scream for a break. Those are the players of that Adidas shoe commercial that asks, "Will that player be you?"

THE CONCEPT OF DELIBERATE PRACTICE

What good coaches know from experience is backed up by a wealth of excellent research. Psychologists the world over have studied the best of the best—musicians, artists, typists, athletes, chess players, dancers, pilots, mathematicians, and more—and have found that one trait is common to them all: *they practice*. Deliberate practice. Commit to practice, and performance will follow. What does the military say? "The more you sweat in training, the less you bleed in battle."

Just what is deliberate practice? Dr. Anders Ericsson of Florida State University has been studying this concept for years. He and others define "deliberate practice" as training that is not inherently enjoyable. Playing a sport just for fun is just that—fun. But deliberate practice is directed practice with a definite goal. David Beckham, for example, is known for his free kicks. After team training, he practices free kick after free kick after free kick—just him, the ball, goal, and a movable wall. He practices well after his teammates have showered and left the ground. Like the movie title says, "Nobody bends it like Beckham" (though the Brazilians might debate that statement). That kind of skill is not genetic; it is from deliberate practice and a lot of it. You want to learn to kick with your weak foot? Better find a wall and set aside time, lots of time.

Now just how much practice is needed? Dr. Ericsson's work and the work of many others have shown that the truly elite performers have put in around 10 years and 10,000 hours of practice in their quest for excellence. It is not just the years and hours; the elite usually began their journey at a young age. If one starts later, like in high school or college, and puts in the time, his or her performance will never equal that of those who began young. This doesn't necessarily mean that kids should start specializing at an early age. The best played many

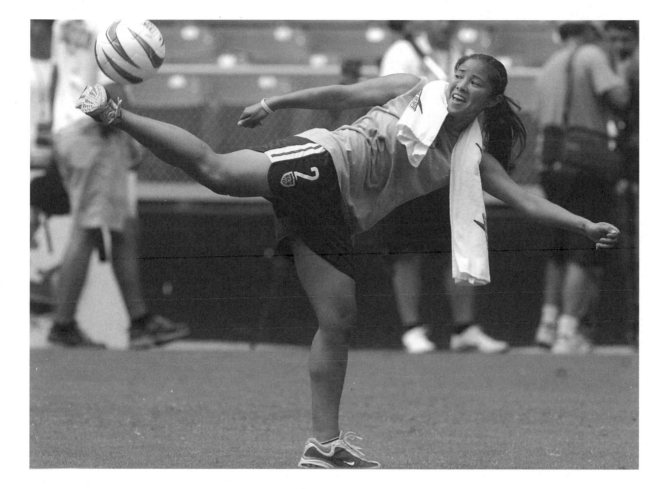

sports and narrowed their focus as they grew more successful and then committed to one sport. Carla Overbeck, the captain of the U.S. women's team when it won the 1996 Olympic gold medal and the 1999 Women's World Cup, was a part of that small class of elite defenders; yet, growing up, she played softball, volleyball, and basketball along with soccer.

Now 10 years and 10,000 hours may sound like an impossible goal. Do the math, and it *is* challenging. Ten years and 10,000 hours averages out to 1,000 hours a year. Divide that by 50 weeks, and you get 20 hours a week, or 3–4 hours a day. This is not as much as a full-time, 40-hour-a-week job, and yet it is obviously not what most kids can give. The professionals spend many hours a day, on the field and off, in preparation. As kids, Pelé, Ronaldo, Zinedine Zidane, and other greats played games for hours in the streets and parks, and that obviously

Practice session before the 2004 Major League Soccer All-Star Game. There is always time to practice your skills. (Photograph by Tony Quinn; SoccerStock.com)

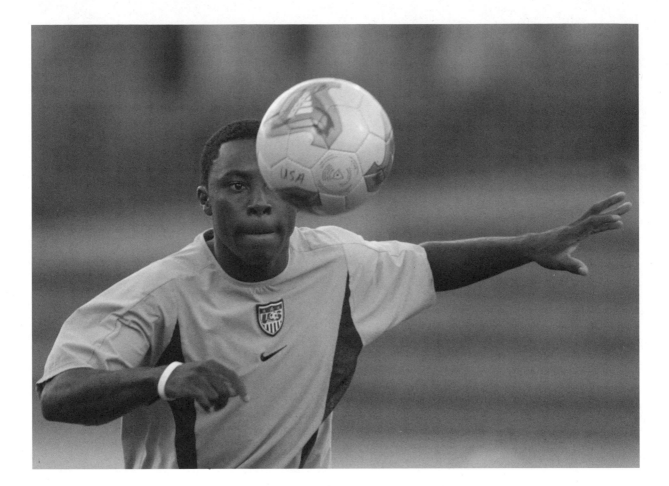

Freddy Adu, 2003 World Championship between the United States and Spain. Concentration on skills and tactics is a key to success. (Photograph by Tony Quinn; SoccerStock.com)

counted. They didn't play just for fun; they played to get better. Bobby Fischer didn't compete at chess all the time, but he was a voracious reader about chess and studied accounts of prior competitions. Danny Karbassiyoon is from the small mountain town of Roanoke, Virginia. In the summer of 2003, he began his professional soccer career on the reserve team of Arsenal FC. I may be wrong, but I bet he spent hours alone, practicing the skills that got him noticed by an Arsenal scout.

I would be the first to say there is more to life than a game. Young players should play different sports and not focus on one sport too early. Unfortunately, the schedules of many current soccer organizations in clubs and schools can limit a player's development if his or her only exposure to the game is through organized practice. A club team may train twice a week for 90 minutes a day and play a game or two on the weekend, for 6–8 hours a week, while schools cram many

INTRODUCTION

games and practices into a very short season. To improve, whether to be a better player or to be one of those truly exceptional players, you will have to put in the time, time alone, time when no one is watching, time away from your team, when the only person driving you is you. If you want to be a better player, *you* are the critical element.

Before every international match governed by the Fédération Internationale de Football Association (FIFA), the teams enter the field, usually escorted by children, and line up near the center of the field. Behind the players is a large yellow flag with the insignia of FIFA Fair Play, easily visible to spectators, television cameras, and photographers.

No doubt, many see this as just a slogan on a flag. On one of my trips to FIFA House, the organization's headquarters in Zurich, I saw how the Fair Play motto extends to virtually every aspect of the game and gives foundation to the game at all levels. As FIFA sources continually attest, "It is FIFA's mission to ensure that the good image of football is always maintained throughout the world. Special attention is paid to promoting the concept of *Fair Play*, with a world-wide campaign aimed at education and ethical values, including the fight against racism and attempted corruption in football."

These are very lofty goals, and to meet these goals FIFA has articulated ten statements of fair play. These concepts are not mutually exclusive; they are interconnected in every aspect at every level of the game. You can't pick and choose. For the good of the game, everyone connected to soccer is obligated to abide by them all. You will see repeated references to Fair Play throughout this book.

1 *Play fair.* An obvious consideration but one that is often ignored. Who hasn't seen a player's jersey pulled? The professional foul? A player writhing on the ground? A dive in the penalty area?
2 *Play to win.* Again, this might seem obvious, but under certain circumstances one or more players on a team might not be trying to win. For example, a team may play for a tie, and sometimes it looks like that right from the opening whistle. But FIFA implores players to always play to win. Anything less shows disrespect to the game.

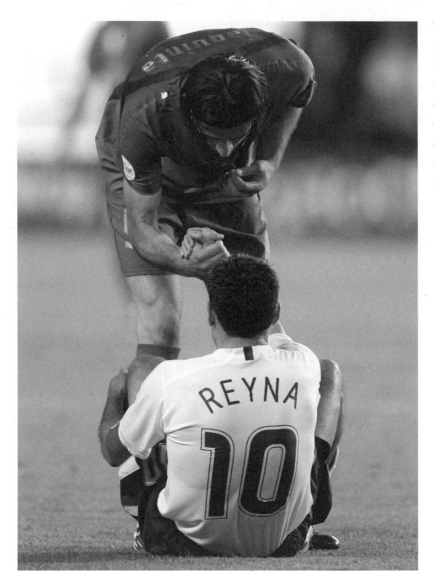

Vincenzo Iaquinta and Claudio Reyna, 2006 FIFA World Cup between the United States and Italy. Half of all injuries to males are due to foul play. Good sportsmanship and fair play will make the game safer and more enjoyable for players and spectators alike. (Photograph by Tony Quinn; SoccerStock.com)

3 *Observe the laws of the game.* Play within the laws as they are set down, and don't try to stretch an interpretation. In an under-10 game, I watched as five players stood, fingertip to fingertip, across the top of the penalty box forming a gauntlet for the other team's goal kick. For this age, it can be quite a challenge for a goal kick to clear the box. Yes, this team observed the laws, but it ignored the statement against unsporting conduct. To the referee's credit, he warned the team, and the second time he gave the coach a yellow card (which was vigorously protested). Because

no 9-year-old would have thought that formation up on his own, the referee carded the guilty party. The team stopped putting up the barrier.

4 *Respect opponents, teammates, referees, officials, and spectators.* Disrespect of fans, teammates, and opponents is seen far too often. One player spits at another. Another player gestures at the ref once the ref turns away. Referees have been given the authority to card or eject players who curse the ref.

5 *Promote the interests of football.* If it is good for the game, within these ten guidelines, then promote these interests.

6 *Honor those who defend football's good reputation.* This begins with your teammates and extends to parents, coaches, referees, and local, state, national, and international administrators. It's the only game the world plays, and it is our duty to protect it.

7 *Reject corruption, drugs, racism, violence, and other dangers to our sport.* Thankfully, the issue of corruption is rare, although not unheard of (the 2005–6 Italian Serie A scandal comes to mind). For the most part, soccer has been pretty resistant to drug use when compared with other major sports like cycling, cross-country skiing, American football, baseball, and ice hockey, but racism and violence are still problems, particularly in the stands. Fortunately, the issue of racism is a front-page topic in Europe now, and governing bodies are coming down hard on clubs whose fans use racist epithets, chants, cheers, flags, and songs.

8 *Help others to resist corrupting pressures.* The financial state of the game is somewhat precarious in some countries, and there might be outside pressures that could damage the game. It is everyone's responsibility to keep corruption out of the game.

9 *Denounce those who attempt to discredit our sport.* In the United States the people who denounce our sport are usually uninformed media out to make some waves and sell some papers. Prior to the 1994 World Cup, which took place in the United States, the media published surveys that said two-thirds of the country didn't even know it was being held. What was their point? That just meant there were 80–90 million people who did! The attendance figures from 1994 probably won't be topped until the World Cup returns to the United States. Do you realize that in 2002, the United States was the second-largest country (after

China) participating in the World Cup with the second-largest number of players (after Brazil)? Speak your mind and defend our sport without taking the defensive stance that the antisoccer media loves.

10 *Use football to make a better world.* Soccer is universal and part of the social fabric worldwide. The sport has the power to impact many facets of life, to promote peace, health, and equality.

CHAPTER 1

Nutrition & Fluid Intake

One of the most influential exercise physiologists in the United States is Dr. David Costill, recently retired from Ball State University in Indiana. He built his academic career around the study of fluid intake and nutritional support for exercise, and many of his students have carried on in his footsteps. After genetics and training, Dr. Costill would say that the most important factor in determining the performance of an athlete is nutrition. His teachings and research have changed the way that individual sport athletes (such as cyclists, runners, swimmers, cross-country skiers, etc.) eat before, during, and after training and competition. Throughout his career, Dr. Costill stressed there is one fundamental difference between what an athlete eats and what a nonathlete eats: volume. Eating a diet that follows the typical recommended daily allowance (RDA) guidelines (see <www.mypyramid.gov>) is all that is needed; an athlete just needs to eat more because training requires more energy from food. Unfortunately, team sport participants have been far less concerned about diet, in spite of a mounting pile of evidence that shows diet can and does affect physical performance.

Much has been written about diet. Large sections of bookstores are devoted to nutrition. Obesity-related disorders may soon eclipse cardiovascular diseases as the main factor in health complications and premature death. Just remember that food intake serves a very simple purpose: providing energy (fuel) for all metabolic processes (outlined in chapter 2). Nutrition and physical activity have been linked for centuries by superstition, tradition, culture, and hearsay. Today it is very common to see a wide variety of food selection in preparation for sport. But regardless of the culture or tradition, the basic building blocks of nutrition are the same worldwide: carbohydrates, fats, proteins, water, vitamins, and minerals. In September 2005 an International Consensus Conference on Nutrition for Football was held at FIFA House. Scientific justification of much of the information in this chapter is based on that conference and can be found at most university libraries in the *Journal of Sports Sciences* July 2006 issue. (A lay summary was produced by FIFA and is available online at <http://www.fifa.com/documents/fifa/medical/Nutrition_Booklet_E.pdf>.)

These drawings show the structure of two simple sugars. When combined, they form sucrose—common table sugar. Glucose is the form in which sugars circulate in the blood. Fructose is the structure of the sugar found in fruits.

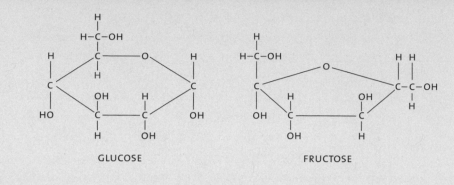

GLUCOSE   FRUCTOSE

CHEMICAL STRUCTURE OF A FAT

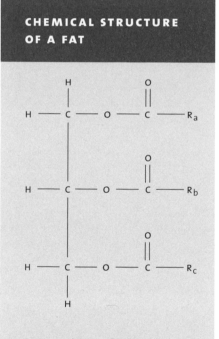

R_a, R_b, and R_c are fatty acid chains of 14–18 carbons in length. Fats differ according to the length and saturation of these fatty acid chains.

- *Carbohydrates*: This is a fundamental source of energy consisting of simple sugars (single or paired molecules like glucose) all the way up to complex chains of multiple sugars (starches). Carbohydrates make up an available, but limited, source of energy for physical activity. They are stored in many areas of the body, most importantly in the liver and muscles, with the latter being the largest location for stored carbohydrates. Stored carbohydrate is called "glycogen." The numerous sprints in soccer place a great demand on stored glycogen. Running out of muscle glycogen is a common reason for fatigue in sports that have an endurance component, like soccer. The best sources of carbohydrates are fruits, vegetables, pasta, cereal, breads, and dairy products.
- *Fats*: The fundamental molecule of fat is called a triglyceride: a glycerol head with three fatty acid chains attached to it. Fats differ according to the length of each chain and whether each carbon in the chain has hydrogen molecules attached (called a saturated fat, which is solid at room temperature, like lard) or does not (called an unsaturated fat, which is a liquid at room temperature, like olive oil). Unsaturated fat is preferred. Fat has a bad reputation because of its connection with heart disease, cancer, obesity, and more. Fat is, however, pretty important and is found around nerves, in muscles, in the blood, packing organs, and under the skin. Fat's bad reputation comes from the type and amount of fat in the blood, under the skin, and elsewhere. Fat is an important energy source

ENERGY CAPACITY IN THE BODY

Organ	Energy
Liver	~400 kilocalories
Skeletal muscle	~2,000–2,500 kilocalories
Adipose tissue	greater than 50,000 kilocalories

and is essentially an inexhaustible supply of energy. The problem is that fat can not supply energy as fast as carbohydrates and can not support the energy requirements of even moderate exercise intensities, only lower intensities. Training improves the body's ability to use fat as a fuel, thus saving carbohydrates. When selecting foods, tropical oils (palm oil, coconut oil, etc.) and trans fats should be avoided. Sources of fat include animal meats, dairy products, nuts, oils, and butter/margarine.

• *Proteins*: The structural building blocks of all cells are proteins. Proteins are also the basis for enzymes, hormones, the chemicals that transmit information between cells, and much more. Most people agree that proteins are a potential, but minor, source of energy during exercise in normal healthy individuals. While most athletes do probably need a little more protein than the spectators, the regular diet of most players is adequate. Protein sources include meats, dairy products, fish, nuts, and beans.

• *Water*: The most common element in the body is also its most important. Water is essential for almost all activities of the cells. For everyone, including the athlete, water is a critical factor in controlling body temperature.

• *Vitamins*: Vitamins are important for a variety of bodily functions; chemical reactions operate more efficiently or more quickly in the presence of specific vitamins. For example, normal blood clotting occurs in the presence of vitamin K, but blood fails to clot in its absence. In addition, selected vitamins (A, E, and C) serve as antioxidants, which can minimize damage and help speed cellular repair.

• *Minerals*: The most common minerals are sodium and chloride (as

Good fat versus bad fat; good carbs versus bad carbs; high carbs versus high protein—it's enough to make you throw your hands up and say, "I give!" What's the deal on each of these?

Good fat versus bad fat: Initially, it was cholesterol that caused concern; people were advised to reduce their cholesterol intake. Cholesterol is the sum total of three different cholesterol molecules—high density, low density, and very low density. It turns out that an elevated level of high-density lipoproteins (HDL) is protective against heart disease, while elevated levels of low-density lipoproteins (LDL) put the person at a higher risk for heart disease. Now trans-fatty acids are the cause for concern. These appear in the diet where different foods are put together to make a product. Most things that come in a wrapper (candy, breakfast bars, cookies, some cereals, and so forth) contain partially hydrogenated fats. These are liquids (oils) that have had hydrogens added to make them more solid. These fats are used sort of like glue, to hold different things together. Natural foods (make sure to study food labels on anything labeled "natural") do not contain trans fats. High amounts of trans fats in the diet are implicated in heart disease. The next iteration of nutrition labels on all foods will have the amount of trans fat in the product.

Good carbs versus bad carbs: Carbohydrates are grouped according to their insulin response. High glycemic foods lead to a rapid and high insulin response, while low glycemic foods elicit a slow and lower insulin response. Now, insulin has a number of roles in the body, but a main one is to help get glucose out of the blood and into the cells. The current thinking

is that a meal of high glycemic foods raises the blood sugar fast, then the insulin response causes the blood glucose to plummet—low blood sugar is a stimulus for hunger, therefore you eat sooner. There are other factors. For example, both white bread and carrots are high glycemic foods. The bread, however, has far more carbs than carrots. So, can you lump all high glycemic foods together? Will the nutrition gurus make up a new factor combining the glycemic index and the grams of carbs in everything? If you weren't confused before, you probably are now. Most research and clinical nutritionists do not feel there is any data to support this concept, even though numerous books have been written on the subject. Athletes eat low or high glycemic foods depending on how fast they want the carbs, as discussed in the text.

High carbs versus high protein: The debate can be heard around the office, the lunch room, the coffee shop, the stands: the relative merits of a high-carb diet (60+% carbs, ~25% fat, ~15% protein) versus a high-protein diet (40-30-30, respectively). The premise of the high-protein diet is that the low intake of carbohydrates leads to less insulin being produced and less carbohydrate stored; thus, the body uses fat as a fuel, and voilà! You lose fat and weight. These diets are under intense scrutiny, but remember one thing: soccer is fueled by carbs. It makes no sense to restrict the soccer player's carbohydrate intake. No sports nutritionist will say that the high-protein diet is good for the competitive athlete. Why do people lose weight on a high-protein diet? Part of the reason is biochemical. Glucose molecules are linked together in cells by a water molecule. With limited carbohydrate intake, the body uses its stored carbohydrate. When glycogen is broken down, a water molecule is split out. Thus the initial weight loss is water. Then, the constant attention paid to one's food intake will keep the person far more aware of what he or she is eating; thus, one will eat only the total calories prescribed instead of snacking, where calories can sneak in.

salt) and potassium. These are necessary for nerves and muscles to function, but they also serve many uses in all cells. Other important minerals include magnesium and calcium.

Every parent and player needs to know that *all* the nutrients needed by the body can be supplied by the normal diet, *if* food choices are made from a wide variety of food sources. A favorite statement of nutritionists is that eating a colorful diet ensures that you are getting almost all the nutrients one needs. Supplementing vitamins and other nutrients with powders, pills, and shakes is unnecessary if athletes choose foods from the variety of sources available. The soccer player's choice of foods should emphasize carbohydrates.

FUEL FOR SOCCER

Energy must be available for running, jumping, shooting, tackling, chasing, dribbling, and other high-intensity activities of the game. Energy must also be available for the lower-intensity parts of the game, like walking and jogging. The fuel for these lower-intensity portions of the game is not as quickly available as is the fuel for the higher-intensity parts. A car has one fuel tank and one fuel, but the body has multiple tanks and different fuels. The body uses carbohydrates for the high-intensity parts of the game that require energy fast and fats for lower-intensity walking and jogging. Because there is a limited amount of carbohydrate stored in the body, training teaches the body to use fat for higher and higher intensities, effectively saving carbohydrates for the highest intensities of work. Research on soccer has shown that as stored glycogen declines throughout a match, the player fatigues, which means that the player runs slower, makes shorter and less frequent runs at higher intensities, executes

FIGURE 1.1

Muscle Glycogen Responses
to Soccer Match Play

Source: Adapted from B. Ekblom,
"Applied Physiology of Soccer,"
Sports Medicine 3, no. 1 (1986):
50–60.

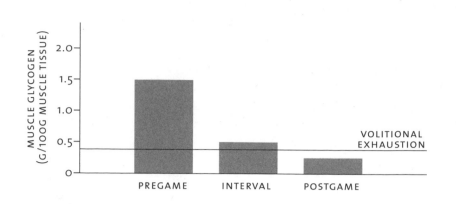

skilled moves poorly, and makes poorer decisions, all at that critical, late period of the game when goals are scored and injuries mount up (figure 1.1).

When you run, you use up fuel, at a rate that depends on the speed of running. Depleted glycogen as the game nears its end is one reason for fatigue in soccer. When an athlete runs out of muscle glycogen, he or she must rely on fat for fuel. The problem is that getting energy from fat is a far slower process than getting energy from carbohydrates, meaning that the athlete can't run as fast when fat is the source of the energy. In fact, when fat is the sole fuel for exercise, the fastest an athlete can run is about 50% of one's ability. Thus, the glycogen-depleted athlete walks or trots.

Figure 1.1 shows the level of muscle glycogen in the legs of soccer players before the game, at halftime, and at the end of the game. The level of glycogen for players before the game is about the same as that of the spectators (you'll have to take my word on this). (One of the things that Costill and many others have shown is that the trained athlete who is in fact eating properly should have *substantially* more muscle glycogen than an untrained spectator.) The muscles use a lot of glycogen in the first half of the game. (Pop quiz: in which half do the players run more? First half. Why? More available fuel.) The final levels of glycogen are low at the end of the game, near zero. Research has shown that once glycogen gets below some level, the athlete will stop voluntary exercise (something one can't really do in a match). This point is called "volitional exhaustion," and the postgame levels of glycogen in the soccer player are *below* this level.

More recent findings relate to the replenishment of muscle glycogen. Research on endurance athletes (such as runners or cyclists) has shown that it takes about 48 hours to fully replenish muscle glycogen after a depleting exercise. Early research on intermittent exercise showed that only 24 hours were needed to replenish glycogen. Later, it was shown that people who did glycogen-depleting eccentric exercise (jumping is a concentric exercise; landing from the jump is an eccentric exercise) took far longer to replenish glycogen. Soccer is not like running straight ahead on a treadmill, as it requires lots of eccentric work—slowing down, stopping, landing, changing directions. The most recent work shows that even in the presence of a high carbohydrate diet, glycogen replenishment can take three or more days. This obviously means that leagues that arrange matches on a Thursday/ Saturday (or similar) schedule are asking players to compete in a less than optimal state, which could lead to reduced performance and greater incidence of injury. The current data, however, do not show greater injury rates in the "second game," probably because the players are playing at a reduced pace due to their low fuel reserves.

Training helps delay fatigue, and there are strategies to help deal with the loss of muscle glycogen. For the player, the goal of training and nutrition is to become so fit that your opponents fatigue first. If they are tired and you aren't, your chances of scoring and avoiding injuries improve.

Proper nutrition is not just about games. Glycogen loss is also a problem in training. For example, say a player eats a typical Western diet (about 40% carbohydrates, 40% fat, and 20% protein) and trains for an hour each day. As a result, he uses up some of his muscle glycogen. Now, it's time to go to the fuel pump—a meal. If his diet does not contain enough carbohydrates to replace the glycogen he used while training, then each day his muscle glycogen levels will stair-step down. If you know an athletic trainer from a high school, college, or professional team, ask when injuries occur, especially during preseason, and he or she will probably say late in the week, as players tire. If the player would eat the diet more commonly recommended for athletes, consisting of 65% or more carbohydrates, 20–25% fat, and 10–15% protein (which is, in fact, *the basic RDA diet!*), muscle glycogen levels can be replaced between workouts. Training causes a partial reduction in glycogen, but sufficient carbohydrates can be eaten to replace the glycogen used (figure 1.2).

This mixture of nutrients is not magic. It's the diet that would be rec-

FIGURE 1.2

Muscle Glycogen Responses
to Three Days of Exercise on a
"Normal" Diet and on the RDA Diet

Source: Adapted from D. L. Costill et al.,
"Muscle Glycogen Utilization during
Prolonged Exercise on Successive Days,"
Journal of Applied Physiology 31, no. 6
(1971): 834–38.

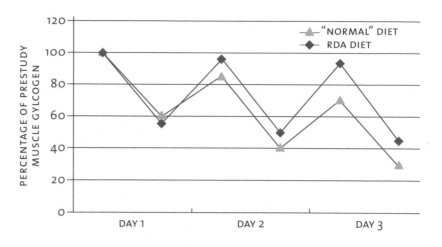

CALORIES, CARBS, AND MACRONUTRIENT MIXTURE

An athlete who eats 3,000 calories a day on the typical Western diet will eat 240 grams of carbohydrate. The player who eats an RDA diet will eat 360 grams of carbohydrate per day. For the first player to eat 360 grams of carbohydrate a day using his current food selections will require 4,500 calories a day.

	Western Diet (3,000 Calories/Day)		
	% of Diet	Calories/Day	Grams/Day
Carbohydrate	40	1,200	240
Fat	40	1,200	133
Protein	20	600	120
	RDA Diet (3,000 Calories/Day)		
Carbohydrate	60	1,800	360
Fat	25	750	83
Protein	15	450	90
	Western Diet (4,500 Calories/Day)		
Carbohydrate	40	1,800	360
Fat	40	1,800	200
Protein	20	900	180

ommended for any healthy individual. The main difference between the preferred diet of an athlete and the preferred diet of a healthy individual is simply the volume of food eaten: eating more supports the additional energy of training and competition. The training athlete who is losing weight during the season (and doesn't want to) needs to increase his food intake. A word of caution: during the season is *not* the time to be trying to gain or lose weight.

Food intake around a match can be divided into the days prior to and after the match and game-day nutrition (prematch, during match, and postmatch).

Days Prior to the Match

The earliest dietary guideline for athletes who wanted to increase the glycogen stored in their muscles was to continue training and limit carbohydrate intake for 3–5 days before competition, then reduce training and increase carbohydrate intake on the last couple of days before competition. The muscles, then, actually would store *more* carbohydrates than normal in the days just before the match. This was a very important advance in sports nutrition. The problem was that training while limiting carbohydrate intake was hard to do, and athletes who followed this advice felt like they were declining right before a competition. Later research showed that to deposit more carbohydrates in muscle all that was needed was to reduce training intensity (assuming the diet was already 65% or more carbohydrates). Most athletes will end up storing up to 50% more fuel (as carbohydrates) in their muscles. Does this allow players to run faster? Not really, but they will maintain their running speed for longer before slowing down. That means they will be running at their early game speed later in the game than their poorly fed opponents. This is a huge plus.

I was part of a survey on suburban high school athletes a few years ago and was surprised to see that athletes ate nearly one meal a day that was delivered to them in a bag (i.e., fast food). In general, soccer players do not choose the best food, meaning their prematch muscle

Ever wonder just what is meant by a "serving"? Nutrition labels on all food containers mention what the serving size is and how many servings the package contains. Ounces, milligrams, milliliters, pounds — but you have no idea what that portion in front of you really is. Here are some quick "conversions" to use when looking at food:

Cereal/pasta: A closed fist is about two standard servings.

Meat/poultry/fish: One serving is about the size of a basic computer mouse or a deck of cards.

Fruit: One medium-sized piece of fruit is about the size of a tennis ball.

Cheese/dairy: One serving of milk is 1 cup, but one serving of cheese is about the size of a pair of dice.

Fat: One serving is 1 ounce of butter (a pat of butter). Or, to put it another way, one serving of fat is the size of the pad of your thumb.

glycogen is not as high as it could be. The relationship between carbohydrates eaten and glycogen stored has been known for over 30 years. The more carbs eaten, the more glycogen stored. Not all players have the nutritional watchdogs that Manchester United, Real Madrid, São Paulo FC, or Juventus might have on salary. The soccer masses (meaning the nonprofessionals) of the world are either not getting the message or not paying attention to the message. In terms of fuel, many players are about as prepared for a match as the spectators.

Game-Day Nutrition

Pregame nutrition. Most athletes should eat a meal about 3–4 hours before competition. The best meal is one that is easily digestible (protein and fat intake slow digestion). Moderate to high glycemic foods, like fruits, cereals, breads, starches (rice, potatoes, noodles, pasta), jellies, and jams, are good options. When carbohydrates are counted (and they should be), 250 or more grams should be eaten.

Within the hour prior to the match, some athletes choose to eat a small amount, 50–100 grams, of (low to moderate glycemic index) carbohydrates. Sports bars and commercial sports drinks (particularly high-carbohydrate drinks) are good options. Doing this increases the blood sugar a little, offering the muscle an alternative source of carbohydrates. In times past, the thinking was that this would cause an insulin response, lowering blood sugar and making the player less alert. This concept, however, has been proven false.

During-game nutrition. The more you run, the more fuel you use, which gradually reduces stored glycogen. During the game, the athlete can ingest a little carbohydrate by drinking some of the newer commercial high-carbohydrate drinks (which are *not* the same as fluid-electrolyte replacement drinks). These drinks have a carbohydrate source that is absorbed so quickly that blood sugar rises within about 5 minutes, giving an alternate source of fuel during activity. Players who use such drinks (before the game and at halftime) could run farther and faster in the second half than players who did not use the drink. In the mid-1970s it was shown that teams using a "glucose syrup" had more ball contacts and shots and goals (especially later in the game) and allowed fewer shots and goals than did the opponents who did not use the syrup. These drinks are *not* a substitute for commercial fluid replacement drinks or water. Carbohydrate replacement

The glycemic index is a statement on the effect of carbohydrates on blood glucose. High glycemic foods bring about a fast rise in blood sugar, which will lead to elevated insulin levels from the pancreas. Insulin then helps transport glucose across cell membranes; this is a very important process after exercise when the body is trying to replenish muscle glycogen. So, during recovery from exercise, it is important to eat high glycemic foods. Eating low and moderate glycemic foods does not elevate blood glucose (and insulin) as much, meaning the slower replenishment of muscle glycogen. What do you see players eating after a game?

High Glycemic Foods	Moderate Glycemic Foods	Low Glycemic Foods
Bagels	Baked beans	Apples
Baked potatoes	Bananas	Chickpeas
Sandwich bread	Bran cereals	Ice cream
Corn syrup	Corn	Beans
Honey	Grapes	Lentils
Maple syrup	Oatmeal	Milk
Raisins	Orange juice	Peanuts
Rice	Pasta	Tomato soup
Chex mix*	Watermelon	Yogurt
Sports drinks	Potato chips	Dates and figs

*Only the ingredients—do not add oil and bake or buy the ready-to-eat mix.

drinks and fluid-electrolyte drinks are two distinctly different products with different uses.

Postgame nutrition. Right after the game is the time to get an early start on putting glycogen back into the muscles. It seems to make some sense that immediately after exercise is when the muscle is most ready to store fuel. So, in the first 1–2 hours after a match (or training), it is important to get some carbohydrates into the body. Plus, there is new information suggesting that a small amount of protein (4 to 1 ratio of carbohydrates to protein) helps speed the uptake of carbohydrates by the muscle, and there are new drinks with this formula. Pay attention to those labels.

CARBS PLUS
BLOOD SUGAR

Carbs are eventually broken down to simple sugars. These differ in how quickly they are absorbed and the eventual amount of glucose that gets into the blood. High glycemic food may yield quick absorption of carbs and a more rapid rise in blood glucose.

COMPARING SPORTS DRINKS

There are two types of sports drinks: fluid and electrolyte replacement versus high carbohydrate. The fluid and electrolyte replacement drinks are primarily used for rehydration and the replacement of salts lost through sweat. High-carbohydrate drinks supply fuel for exercise, and they are used as a fuel alternative or as an initial source of carbohydrates right after exercise. The two types of drinks are not interchangeable. During exercise, players will likely want to drink water or a commercial replacement drink. Both should be made available. The reason for having both is that most players will, on their own, create a mix that closely matches their own peculiar sweat. Those whose sweat is dilute (not very salty) will probably choose to consume more water, while those who sweat a highly salty sweat will favor the commercial drink. (Professional teams hire people to analyze the sweat of their players and develop a specific, individual recipe for each player.) Right before the game, at halftime, and right after the game, players should have a high-carbohydrate drink available.

Some parents get confused when reading the labels on commercial drinks or the powders that are mixed with water. A major difference between drinks is the carbohydrate source.

Maltodextrins: These are a string of glucose molecules, usually six or seven bound together. A subject of intense study, maltodextrins get out of the stomach and intestines and into the blood very quickly—often within 5 minutes. A factor in solutions is osmolarity, which is related to the number of particles in solution, not to the size of particles. One string of a maltodextrin and one glucose molecule contribute equally to the osmolarity. The glucose molecule, however, only contributes one molecule of glucose, while the maltodextrin eventually contributes six to seven molecules of glucose. Not only do maltodextrins get into the blood fast, but they also contribute more fuel, making them the carbohydrate of choice for drinks.

Fructose: This is the structure of carbohydrates in fruit. Typically, fructose is not the primary source of carbohydrates. On a label, fructose will likely be the third or fourth ingredient listed (ingredients are listed in order from most to least). The problem is that fructose is not all that easily absorbed through the intestine, and then it must go to the liver to be converted to glucose for use by muscle. One might as well use straight glucose and avoid the extra step. However, fructose is commonly used to improve the taste of the drink, as glucose isn't all that tasty.

Sucrose: This is simple table sugar and is one part glucose and one part fructose. For use as energy, it first must be split in two, and then the fructose must be converted into glucose. Like fructose, sucrose is not likely to be the first carbohydrate listed.

Galactose: You might find the labels of drinks with galactose claiming better performance. Galactose is derived from lactose, the sugar in milk. While galactose is fairly effective at maintaining blood sugar, no study has ever shown it to improve performance—the outcome of interest.

Polylactate: Some drinks tout polylactate as a performance aid. This is a carbohydrate with an amino acid (often arginine) attached. The first study on its use was favorable, but no subsequent research has shown it to have any benefit at all.

Not many players want to sit down to a meal right after a game. So, the player needs to make the best food choices. A good start are the commercial high-carbohydrate drinks just mentioned, especially those 4 to 1 ratio carb/protein drinks. Drinks like these can be found in better specialty sports (especially cycling) stores or nutrition stores. Moderate to high glycemic index foods are prime choices and include fresh or dried fruits, bagels with jam/jelly, or high-carbohydrate cereals eaten dry (e.g., Chex mix ingredients). The athlete should avoid eating very high protein or fatty meals or drinking carbonated beverages. The current thinking is that the carbonation makes the player feel full much sooner, and he or she eats and drinks less as a result. Alcohol is not advised because of the diuretic effect alcohol can have on an already dehydrated player. The goal is to try to take in 50–100 grams of carbohydrate, as well as the corresponding amount of protein (the 4 to 1 ratio would mean 12–25 grams of protein), in the 1–2 hours after the match. I just hang my head when I wander around youth soccer matches and see the ubiquitous cooler come out, the kids flocking for a juice box and a bag of chips.

Over the rest of the 24-hour day, the player needs to select foods high in (low to moderate glycemic index) carbohydrates to take in about 7–10 grams per kilogram of body weight. The 70 kilogram (154 pound) player would try to eat between 500 and 700 grams of carbohydrate in 24 hours. This takes planning. No one eats this much carbohydrate at one meal. A 1-pound box of dry spaghetti has eight servings, and each serving has 42 grams of carbohydrate. So that one box has 336 grams of carbohydrate in it. To get 500 grams of carbohydrate by eating spaghetti would require 1.5 *pounds* of dry spaghetti! Go ahead, I dare you. Cook it up and see just how much that is. As a result, you have to plan to get carbs from different sources and spread out your eating throughout the day.

FLUIDS

By now, it should be common knowledge that during exercise fluids must be consumed in order to delay dehydration and prevent heat illness. I can remember when withholding water was a common practice. It is quite possible that a coach today who withholds water during training could find himself in a position of negligence should water restriction lead to a medical problem.

Why is water so important? The work done by muscles produces heat that must be eliminated. There are four ways for the body to rid itself of heat: radiant heat loss, conductive heat loss, convective heat loss, and—the most important method during exercise—evaporation. These will be discussed in more detail in chapter 2. Just remember that sweating is not heat loss: evaporation of sweat is heat loss. The longer the duration of exercise and the greater the evaporation of sweat, the less the total amount of water in the body, meaning less water for the control of body temperature, and body temperature will increase.

Why is this so important? In the absence of water during exercise, the core body temperature rises; drinking water during exercise keeps the body temperature from rising (figure 1.3). An uncontrolled rise in body temperature can lead to heat exhaustion and heatstroke—a medical emergency that can be fatal (remember Korey Stringer of the Minnesota Vikings?). Heat illness is not a trivial situation, and its prevention should be paramount in the minds of people who oversee sports.

In addition, as body water and weight declines, performance also

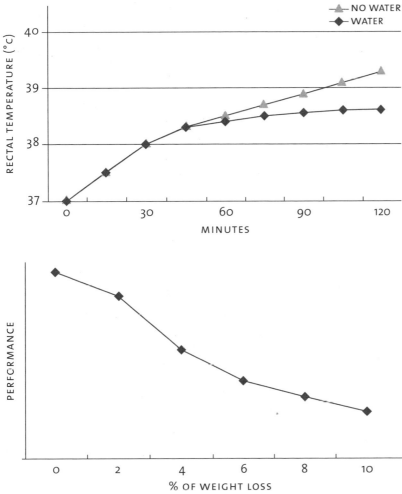

FIGURE 1.3

Core Body Temperature Responses to Exercise with and without Water

Source: Adapted from D. L. Costill et al., "Fluid Ingestion during Distance Running," *Archives of Environmental Health* 21, no. 4 (1970): 520–25.

FIGURE 1.4

Effect on Performance of Increasing Levels of Dehydration

Source: Adapted from R. J. Maughan, "Fluid and Electrolyte Loss and Replacement in Exercise," *Journal of Sports Science* 9 (1991): 117–42.

declines. As little as a loss of 2% of body weight by sweating can lead to lower performance levels. The problem is that the body's thirst mechanism is poor; most people don't even feel thirsty until they have lost 2% of body weight. So, by the time a player feels thirsty, he or she may already be seeing a decline in performance in the physical, mental, technical, and tactical domains (figure 1.4).

The scientific literature has established the recommended levels for drinking water or fluid-electrolyte replacement drinks. Typically, the recommendation is to drink around 500 milliliters (approximately 16 ounces) in the hour prior to exercise, then about 150–250 milliliters (5–8 ounces) of fluids every 15–20 minutes during exercise, trying to get around 750 milliliters to 1 liter (three-quarters to a full quart) per hour. Most players will sweat out more than this during exercise and few will replace sweat lost with fluids ingested on a milliliter for milliliter basis. This is not just for training in hot weather. Training in cool weather still leads to sweat losses of water; however, players tend not to drink the same amount in cool weather that they do in warmer weather.

During training, fluid breaks can be scheduled easily. During a game? Why, soccer is a game of constant activity, no timeouts, it can't be done! Nonsense, soccer has plenty of time when the ball is not in play. The ball is in play for around 60–70 minutes of a 90-minute game. Put water bottles in each goal and along both sidelines, and make water available during injury stoppages, during substitutions, and when the ball is out of play. Some youth developmental leagues have four quarters in a game instead of the traditional two halves. That setup can be good for fluid intake and brief coaching instructions. I've known of summer games changed at kickoff from two halves to four quarters in order to allow a rest period for fluid intake, and of games where each half is shortened and time is added to halftime.

It really is unrealistic to expect any athlete to keep up with water loss by drinking during exercise. Any player who keeps his or her weight lost to 2% or less has done well. So, after a game, the player needs to replenish fluids. The typical formula is about 1.5 liters per kilogram of body mass lost (or about 1.5 pints per pound of weight lost). This can't be done in a single serving, as the volume overload to the stomach might trigger vomiting or diarrhea (been there, done that!). The goal is to be back to the pregame weight within 24 hours. Many clubs require players to weigh themselves before and after practices or games for just this purpose. It's hardly a big deal and doesn't take away from practice time. Assign a parent to bring a scale to training and record weights (privately, if needed).

VITAMINS AND SUPPLEMENTS

Vitamins can be fully replaced in a well-balanced diet that contains plenty of fruits and vegetables (remember, eat a colorful diet). Some of the commercial drinks contain antioxidant vitamins that can help speed tissue repair. The use of a multivitamin that contains electrolytes may be of benefit to players who do not consume a well-balanced

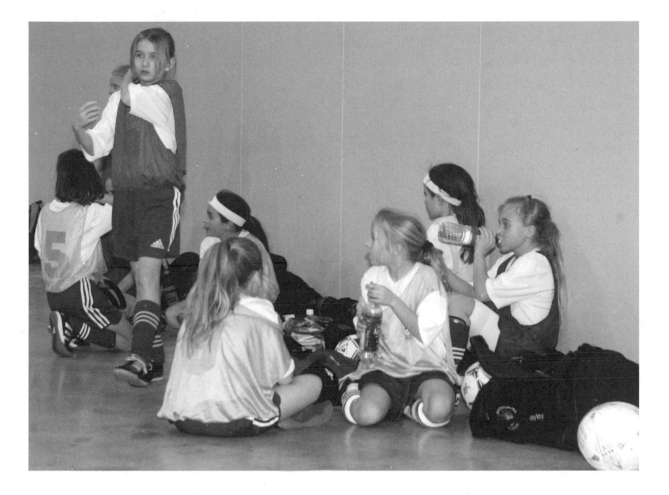

diet, although many athletes take a multivitamin (just to be sure) and there is nothing wrong with that. There is some rationale for postpubertal women to supplement their diet with iron, but only if medically suggested. Reports indicate that on some women's national teams as many as 25% of members need some form of iron supplementation (under a physician's guidance). A nutritionist (a dietician with an R.D., or registered dietician, certification after her name) can be a valuable source of information, especially if she is sports-minded.

The number of supplements on the market is staggering, and many stores specialize in these products. Plus, hundreds of books have been written for a field that changes almost every day. Why do people take supplements? They may say that they are trying to get things in their bodies that they aren't getting from their diet (believe me, it's a whole lot cheaper to get those nutrients from nature instead of a powder

Players need to develop good habits early to minimize dehydration. A regular schedule of drinking during training and matches will keep dehydration at bay. (Photograph by Tony Quinn; SoccerStock.com)

The American College of Sports Medicine (ACSM) is the world's largest professional organization of experts in the exercise sciences. They have prepared and updated the guidelines for fluid replenishment during exercise. Based on the massive amount of research conducted on the topic, ACSM recommends the following:

- Weigh in before exercise.
- Drink 150–200 milliliters of fluids (about one to two good mouthfuls) in the 15–30 minutes prior to exercise.
- Drink 150–200 milliliters of fluids every 15–20 minutes during exercise.
- Weigh out after exercise.
- Replace lost fluids over the next 24 hours at a rate of ingesting 1.5 pints of water for every 1 pound of weight lost.
- Start exercise at the same weight each day.

Practically speaking, it is unlikely that one will replace, ounce for ounce, fluids lost as sweat with fluids ingested during exercise. About the best an athlete can hope to do is minimize fluid loss to less than 2% of body weight.

Other considerations:

- Water can be a little bland, so a drink with some flavor might get athletes to drink more. Teams should supply water and a flavored drink, and let players choose.
- Cold drinks are more palatable than tepid or room temperature drinks.
- The human thirst mechanism is not all that great. Most players have lost 2% of their body weight before they even want to drink anything. You may have to remind them to drink—over and over and over.
- Fluids only work if they stay in the body. Water is very effective. Watch your urine color, and it will lighten up pretty quick but get darker again in a few hours. Drinks with some salt in them stay in the body longer and are even more effective.
- A fluid replenishment drink and a carbohydrate replacement drink are *not* the same thing. One is for fluids, the other for fuel. Both help fend off fatigue but by different mechanisms. Don't confuse one for the other.
- In 2005 there were reports in the popular media about marathon runners drinking too much water during a race, which could lead to a potentially harmful dilution of the blood. Some runners actually gained weight during a run. Soccer doesn't have multiple aid stations, and while there are opportunities for fluids during play, they are limited. I find it hard to believe that a similar situation could exist in soccer, unless some overzealous coach pushed too much water too frequently during training. There are anecdotal reports of some women weighing more after training due to excessive water intake.
- The beer issue: There are nationalistic traditions where beer is supplied in the locker room after a match (been there, done that, too). Beer has been studied for its fluid replenishment properties (the studies were done in Scotland—ask me about the Scottish double century some time). Beer has been supplied to some athletes to start the urine

flow for a drug test after a very hot game. Now, the body is pretty smart. Although alcohol stimulates urine flow, the body says that getting fluids is more important, so the side effect of alcohol on urine flow is suppressed until some level of hydration has been reestablished. Then the urine production begins again. It doesn't start right away with beer ingestion—it takes some time. I know some people who do the drug testing for the World Cup, and they say for some games the stadium is completely empty by the time a player has been able to generate a urine sample. Ask players what they would rather do for doping control after a match—a urine or blood test? They always say blood because they'll get out of doping control quicker.

• After a game or training, stay away from carbonated drinks or overly sweet drinks (like juice boxes). Players tend to feel full too quickly and don't drink as much.

or a pill). Truthfully, most athletes are trying to get an edge over the competition, be it to gain playing time or to beat their opponents. Supplements claim to make you bigger, help with weight loss, make you stronger, help you recover faster, enable you to work harder, longer, and more frequently, and so on. Many supplements are banned from school, college, professional, or international competition, but many others don't make the lists of banned substances. To quote a leading nutrition and exercise researcher, Dr. Ronald Maughan of Loughborough University in England: "If it works, it's probably banned. If it isn't banned, it probably doesn't work." There are few things that one can put in one's mouth that will improve performance beyond those discussed above: carbohydrate intake (as food or high-carbohydrate drinks) and fluid-electrolyte drinks.

One supplement that has been widely used with some success in certain sports is creatine. This helps the body transfer energy during very high-intensity short-term work, but many athletes are "nonresponders" (a player who takes the supplement but gets no effect). The main side effect is rapid weight gain, and the medical community is concerned about potential long-term effects. Some players use it for training, others for matches. Its effectiveness in soccer, however, is still unknown. Why? Because all the research has been on performance in a limited number of sprints (like six), not on the lengthy time and distances covered in soccer. One study on soccer showed creatine "worked," but there are problems with this study. First, only

Any supplement with any of the following ingredients should be avoided. Lists like these are *never* complete, so check with appropriate authorities before taking *any* supplement reported to contain a natural muscle-building substance.

Dehydroepiandrosterone (DHEA)
Androstenedione
Androstendiol
4-Androstenediol
5-Androstenediol
19-Norandrostenedione

Here is an incomplete list of products that could trigger a positive test for nandrolone:

Ingredient	Product
DHEA	Twinlab 7-Ketofuel
	Twinlab Growth Fuel
	Twinlab DHEA Fuel
	Twinlab Tribulus Fuel Stack
	Olympian Labs DHEA
	MuscleTech Anotesten
Androstenedione	Champion Androstendione
	MuscleTech Anotesten
	MuscleTech Nortestin
	Cytodyne Androdyne
	Olympian Labs Androstene Power
	Twinlab 7-Ketofuel
Androstenediol	ASN Maxabol
	GEN Cyclodex 4-Adiol
	MuscleTech Acetabol ANII
	MuscleTech Anotesten
	Cytodyne Androdyne

a small number of players were studied, which is always a problem in supplement studies. The research design gurus say that a proper supplement study needs to have around 350 subjects, and I defy anyone to find a sport supplement study with that many subjects. Second, it is very difficult to blind subjects to creatine use. Remember, the side effect of creatine use is noticeable, rapid weight gain. In studies like this, subjects are not supposed to know what they are being given, but if their weight rises over only a few days, chances are good that they will think they have been given creatine. Since most already feel that creatine "works," they may try harder. Now, this doesn't mean that creatine isn't being used by soccer players. I've visited professional clubs in numerous countries and have seen bottles of creatine in training rooms. But given the length of soccer games and the problem of carrying around that extra weight, one can question whether creatine has any utility in soccer.

Any player who has the potential of representing his or her country has to be very careful of what he or she ingests. A seemingly harmless supplement or over-the-counter medication may contain precursors to banned substances, leading to a positive drug test. Recently, the World Anti-Doping Agency (WADA) suggested that certain substances found in common over-the-counter cold medicines, as well as caffeine, be removed from the banned list because their influence on performance is negligible. There is little, if any, governmental oversight of the supplement industry and no regulations on truth in labeling. Studies on labeling accuracy show wild variations in what the label says and what the supplement actually contains. Many supplements on the shelves and the Internet make outrageous claims about ingredients that even an organic chemist couldn't decipher. These products could also contain unlisted chemicals that could trigger a positive drug test. Think about it. In a weight-gain product, a company might add some steroid and elect not to indicate it on the label. People buy it because the product works, but it probably worked by means other than what the labeling says. Remember, the supplement industry does not have Food and Drug Administration (FDA) oversight. No sport governing body accepts ignorance as a satisfactory defense. Most national governing bodies of sport work very hard at educating players in their national team pools in an effort to keep their athletes from being stupid and taking something that could trigger a positive drug test. It is practically a full-time job keeping athletes clean.

WHAT ABOUT THE VEGETARIAN PLAYER?

While there are a variety of vegetarian diets, the vegetarian player follows the same nutritional guidelines. In general, the absence of meat in the diet means that other protein sources need to be provided—for example, eggs, cheese, and dairy products. Beans (black, kidney, lima, lentils, etc.) are excellent sources of both protein and insoluble fiber. Add nuts (peanuts, cashews, etc.) and seeds (sunflower, pumpkin, etc.) to a dish, and the vegetarian athlete can get all the protein needed.

The only concern might be the need for some iron, which meat would normally provide. Whole-grain cereals contain iron; the small intestine can better absorb the available iron if the cereal is served with fruit juices (but not coffee, tea, milk, or red wine). Spinach, other leafy greens like kale or mustard greens, and almonds are loaded with iron. In some cases, a physician might suggest an iron supplement. Menstruating female athletes may need to take an iron supplement, upon medical suggestion.

THE "ELITE" PLAYER

An "elite" player has particular needs. The gifted player may play for multiple teams, over a long (or overlapping) season, and train harder and more frequently than most players. He or she may also get more support and advice but nevertheless eat most meals away from the team, which means that the player must take responsibility for food choices.

Nutrition choices before, during, and after game time not only impact league matches but also various tournaments, cups, scrimmages, and more. Fatigue is mostly related to declining muscle glycogen levels, and the more glycogen that is stored, the later fatigue will occur in a match. The intense level of play also leads to more fluid loss, so the elite player must drink when the opportunity presents itself. The player most in need of fluid replenishment is also the hardest person to get to: central midfielders run the most, but they are also the farthest from the sidelines.

Elite players must pay attention to their diet—to watch over practically every meal and food choice—not just before a match but also during training. Training at this level is usually more frequent and intense. Poor refueling can lead to fatigue, poor performance, and injury. The elite player is competing for playing time, and poor nutrition will impact on one's training performance, which could affect selection for the match.

To compensate for these expanded needs, the newly elevated "elite" player (and family) will likely need some special instructions and resources on food choices, intake, and timing. The prematch meal may be a team gathering and guided by a trained sports nutritionist. Fluid needs may be more closely monitored, as players learn how to manage game restrictions and fluid needs. Immediate postmatch nutrition may also be a team function, guided by the team nutritionist or other knowledgeable person. In such cases, food choices will be provided for the player at the appropriate times. Alcohol should be avoided. Remaining meals will probably be the choice of the player; the player should follow club instructions and not fall back into prior, less desirable habits.

Semipro teams usually consist of older players who have played at a higher level and younger players who want to "move up." Older players tend to know what works for them, while younger players want more training for added improvement. This mix is a challenge because of the preconceived habits and practices of those of all ages.

Additional challenges stem from the time constraints of semipro players. Semiprofessional players must balance their work/career schedules with training sessions, which are often in conflict with each other. Training is less frequent and strenuous than that of the elite professional player and usually takes place after the typical workday. This time crunch can make adequate nutrition a challenge. Moreover, support of the team can be quite variable; some get a great deal of help, while others have little, if any, ancillary assistance. Matches tend to be on a fixed, once weekly, schedule. The level of intensity and total volume of work during a match are lower than in elite play, and sometimes games may be scheduled midweek after the normal workday.

Players at this level are unlikely to have access to a club nutritionist and must make their own decisions on choices, volume, and timing of food intake, a difficult process that is further compounded by the sometimes conflicting issues of work and play. For example, the prematch meal for a midweek game would need to be consumed in the afternoon of the workday at a different time than the normal midday meal. Sometimes players live together and should share sound (as opposed to traditional) nutrition information. Weekend matches are more easily handled. (At least match density is lower than at the elite level.) These players, as at all levels, should try to keep dehydration to 2% of body weight lost or less. These players may need to seek out nutritional help on their own.

The vast majority of players worldwide would be considered amateurs, who play for the sheer joy of the game. They may enjoy the level they play at or want to move up a level of competition. The range of ages can be from the very young to older adults. The teams are usually organized around matches and likely don't have any real support other than for scheduling, but there are some sponsored teams that provide some support for their players.

Training the amateur player is very team- and player-specific. Some teams only compete, while others undertake training during one or more sessions a week that focus mostly on technique and tactics, with little emphasis on fitness. As such, dietary concerns for training that are important for the elite or semiprofessional player are not as important. Players should follow normal healthy guidelines (see <www.mypyramid.gov> with respect to the mixture of carbohydrates, fats, and proteins.

The number of competitive matches varies greatly among teams and leagues, but usually games are scheduled once per week. Teams may also sign up for the occasional weekend tourney that could have multiple brief games or two full games in two days. Most matches are played at a slower pace with less overall running as compared with higher levels of play. Many leagues modify the laws to suit their purposes, particularly substitution rules, allowing free substitution throughout the match, which further reduces the volume and intensity of play. Those players who do play 90 minutes might deplete their glycogen, but most, who play less, probably won't use as much stored fuel. Therefore, most amateurs do not need to eat the high volume of carbohydrates recommended for the pros (7–10 grams per kilogram of body weight); 5–7 grams per kilogram should suffice. (This may not hold true for youth players who overcompete by playing on multiple teams, which leads to some playing up to 100 or more matches a year.)

Just because the match and training demands are less strenuous than those at higher levels of play does not mean the amateur can't benefit from following these guidelines. Remember, the main difference between a well-rounded diet and the diet of an athlete is simply the volume eaten by the athlete to support the extra demands of training and competition. The relative mixture of carbs, fats, and proteins is the same; the athlete just eats more. Amateur players will have to pay attention to their own fluid needs, as there is not likely to be someone watching out for them. Sharing fluid bottles is not advised (I've seen pro teams that have had a flu bug run through a team and have learned to number each bottle so that a player drinks only from his or her own bottle). Amateur players should monitor their weight closely to maintain a competitive weight because the season is shorter with longer breaks. Eat less during the breaks (and continue supplemental exercise) to avoid weight gain. The social aspects of adult amateur soccer can involve alcohol, so prudent use is advised.

THE FEMALE PLAYER

While the volume of running in the women's game is around 30% less than the men, the intensity is still around 70% of capacity. Unfortunately, there is little research on women players, so we borrow from work on other women athletes. Players should follow the same concepts as men: eat enough to support training, competition, and everyday activities, as well as a body composition that supports their health and athletic goals. Research on female athletes shows many are in a negative calorie balance: they eat less than they need in an attempt to control weight. This deficit can impact their health and their performance.

The main issues here are pressure and unrealistic goals for the amount of body fat. Low calorie intake leads to fatigue during the day and during sport. The "female athlete triad" is a documented problem in sports and must be considered by all who are associated with females in sports. Chapter 3 deals with the triad.

Losing body fat is difficult and should be looked at as a long-term goal, not a short-term process. Rapid weight loss is usually water loss. The main thing to remember is that during the season is not the time to attempt weight loss. To lose weight requires one to be in a negative calorie balance by limiting calorie intake, and during the season this would limit the energy available for training and competition. It is better to focus on weight loss in the off-season, then try to maintain weight during the season.

Most people, athletes and spectators alike, have unrealistic goals for weight loss. The best way to determine a healthy weight is by having one's body composition measured. This process determines the percentage of the body weight that is fat. Let's say a 150-pound player is 20% fat. That means she has 30 pounds of fat and 120 pounds of everything else. If she wants to get to 15% fat, her goal would be 141 pounds; to get to 10% fat, 133 pounds. By the way, most competitive (not amateur) males are 5–12% fat and, women are 12–20% fat.

Reducing fat is hard, and there is no magic bullet. Reduce portion sizes; don't skip meals or eliminate food choices. Choose healthy (low-fat) snacks wisely, and save some calories from a meal for a later snack, but keep up the carbohydrate intake. Swap high-fat foods for lower-fat options. When preparing food, bake, broil, or boil—don't fry. Limit (or eliminate) alcohol intake. Higher-fiber foods fill one up sooner, and they are of a lower glycemic index, which leads to less of an insulin response.

Some women, under medical advice, may find it necessary to pay attention to their calcium and iron intakes. Calcium (particularly for bones) can be found in calcium-fortified juices and dairy foods. Added calcium is usually suggested during growth, adolescence, pregnancy, and breast-feeding. Low iron is a factor in overall, and sports-related, fatigue. Menstruating females are at a higher risk for iron-related issues. Iron can be found in red meats, iron-fortified breakfast cereals, and deep green vegetables (like spinach). Iron absorption by the intestines is enhanced with vitamin C and some factors found in meats. Iron supplementation (as pills or other supplements) should only be undertaken under a physician's orders.

THE YOUNG PLAYER

I never know what to believe when I hear reports on youth sport participation. During the 2006 FIFA World Cup, I heard that soccer had become the most popular sport in the United States. All these very young players (which I will define as under 10 years of age) have unique nutritional needs during this period of rapid growth.

Youth training and games differ widely from what we see on television. The games are shorter, with different rules, sizes of field, numbers of players, and more. Boys and girls may be on the same teams.

Training is usually about skills and less about fitness or tactics. Training sessions might be two short sessions a week or simply a session right before a match. Some players who show a knack for or an increased interest in the game may start playing on multiple teams or play other sports as well. Certain talented players may even start "playing up" by joining a team with older players.

Competitive games at this level usually follow modified rules, especially as relate to guaranteed participation. The player on multiple teams may play a number of games each week, placing added strain on the energy supply for sport and growth.

A problem is that many coaches are volunteer parents who have little sport background or much idea of where to get information. Leagues and state associations should make resources available for their coaches. This is an ideal time to start children thinking about good food choices, and coaches are well positioned to have some influence, assuming they are knowledgeable and are a good role model. Providing soda pop and chips after a game is not a beneficial example for players to follow.

We have all heard that "children are not little adults," and nowhere is this more evident than in how children deal with the heat. Special considerations must be made for children. This is one reason their games are often played in quarters, rather than halves, to allow some time to rest, get a drink, and cool off. Coaches should also ensure that players have proper clothing to help with heat dissipation—not all T-shirts are created alike. This is also a great time to get children thinking about continuing exercise to be healthy and combat the rising tide of childhood obesity. There is no evidence to suggest that children need any supplements to support, or speed, growth.

The best way to get children to increase their energy intake is by increasing the number of times they eat each day. Five or more small meals are better than three larger meals. Extra energy can come from fruit "smoothies" or milkshakes (note: a "shake" doesn't have enough dairy in it to be called a milkshake, so choose wisely). High-carbohydrate foods (drinks, energy bars) are good sources of quick energy. Most parents would like children to eat less candy, but if candy is desired, the so-called clear candies (gumdrops, jelly beans, "gummy" candy, non-chocolate-based candy; you get the idea) have more carbs, less fat, and fewer overall calories. Children can get plenty of carbohydrates from breakfast cereals and milk, sandwiches made from English muffins or bagels, yogurt, smoothies, fruits, and more.

THE REFEREE

The forgotten person in a match is the referee. Most of the focus is on the players, but the referee is in a position to have an impact on the outcome of a match and should not be ignored. Several studies on the work rate of the referee show that the referee covers about the same distance as the players, but with a little different running pattern (for example, the ref covers more ground going backwards than most field players, jogs more, and sprints less). There is very little in referee education on nutrition, but more emphasis on fitness is now common.

Teams train together, but referees are on their own. The level of play usually dictates how hard and far they run; thus, they need to be prepared for the highest level of play they are likely to work. In other words, referees should follow the same nutritional suggestions as the players whose games they work. The same goes for nutrition before, during, and after a match.

A particular issue is fluids during a match for the referee. Each team may have someone watching out for the players, but the referee may (and "may" is the operative word) have only the fourth official. At lower-level matches, referees may have no one with them. During injury or booking stoppages, uninvolved players may have the chance to drink, but the referee is in the middle of these situations and has no opportunity to drink. In addition, the referee is usually in the middle of the field, far from the sidelines. The referee's assistants are the lucky ones on the sidelines and can place drinks along their running paths. One option for the referee is to wear a small "camelback" like cyclists use. The ref would only need to put a pint to a quart in it and drink when needed, then replenish at halftime. A pint of water is only a pound of weight and wouldn't be a factor in the ref's ability to keep up with play. Another option on particularly hot days would be for the referees and coaches to all agree to take a short break halfway through each period. At a normal stoppage of the game (probably a goal kick or throw in), stop the game, bring drinks out, and then continue where play left off. The referee has the authority to do this, and such a break would be probably be welcomed by players and coaches alike. No game is so important that it can't be interrupted for a minute or two.

PLAYING WHEN TRAVELING

Most highly competitive players travel, sometimes for a few hours, sometimes for days. Even the recreational player will sometimes have to travel to play. Being out of the home environment presents unique challenges for quality nutrition. The normal training routine is upset; the match may be played in a different environment; jet lag and travel fatigue, different local customs (even within the United States), and reliance on "eating out" all can disrupt proper eating. Many teams look for buffets for a wide food selection at a reasonable price, but people can overeat or make poor choices when presented with such an array of foods.

Eating well while traveling can be accomplished by planning ahead. While traveling, realize that long-term exposure to air-conditioned cars or pressurized airplane cabins increases fluid losses, and players need to be encouraged to drink; however, these same players need to be cautioned not to eat out of boredom. Know what to expect at the destination, as plans may have to be made regarding what foods to take and what might need to be obtained at a grocery store. Hotels with food service are usually willing to accommodate the special needs and requests of teams. Traveling in the United States means the local water will probably not cause gastrointestinal upset, but when traveling outside of the United States, it is best to check if bottled water would be advisable. (From personal experience: many Americans like lots of ice in cold drinks. You may be in a place where bottled water is advised, but players forget and get ice added to their drinks, which could lead to problems.) It is probably a good idea to avoid street food, salads, or unpeeled fruit not prepared by a quality restaurant. These foods may give a local experience, but they could have been in contact with local soil and water. Some teams will take a supply of portable foods when traveling like cereals, energy bars, spreads (jam, honey, peanut butter), powdered sports drinks, and dried fruits. Finally, stick to an eating plan (timing and selections) that is close to home practices.

1. Choose a mixture of foods that leads to a diet of about 65% carbohydrates, 20–25% fat, and 10–15% protein. Choosing from a variety of food sources will also help ensure adequate intake of vitamins and minerals. Remember: a colorful diet is best.

2. Choose carbohydrates so that about 7–10 grams/kilogram are eaten over a 24-hour period. Read those labels! The player should also drink plenty of water during this period.

3. Pregame, most athletes like a small carbohydrate meal 3–4 hours prior to kickoff. In the last hour, a high-carbohydrate snack or a high-carbohydrate drink can be consumed.

4. During the game, drink fluids whenever the opportunity occurs. Plastic water bottles should be placed in both goals and along the touch lines, especially during hot and humid weather. During training fluids should be made available every 15–20 minutes, more often if it is really hot.

5. At halftime, a high-carbohydrate drink can help increase second-half running volume and intensity.

6. After the game, take in 50–100 grams of carbohydrate in the first 1–2 hours and also drink fluids to start rehydrating. The goal is to drink about 1.5 liters per kilogram (or 1.5 pints per pound) of body mass to return to normal weight within about 24 hours.

7. With a balanced diet from a variety of food sources, the need for supplements is low. Some women may benefit from a *medically suggested* iron supplement.

8. Most exercise-related claims of supplements are without merit. Whether creatine is beneficial for soccer is unknown.

9. Ingestion of supplements places the potential national team player or collegiate player at risk of a positive drug test because there is little government oversight of the supplement industry. There is no guarantee that the list of ingredients on the label is accurate or truthful.

Training

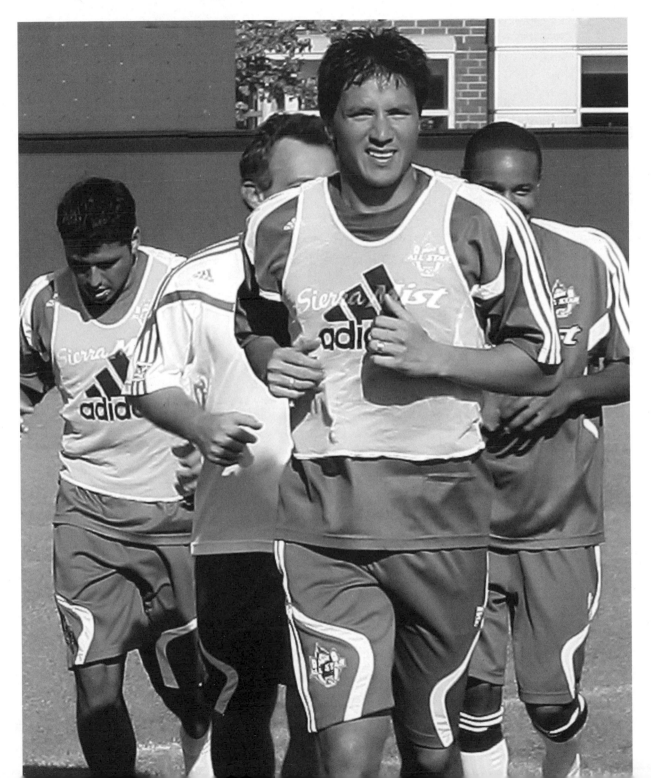

"Physical fitness" is an umbrella term for many factors that influence human physical performance. Some sports, like the marathon, require exceptional whole body endurance, but not much in the way of power output (play basketball with a distance runner some time—and laugh at their poor vertical jump). Other sports, like the 400-meter dash, require a high anaerobic component, speed, strength, and local muscle endurance. American football demands high strength, speed, and power, while gymnasts need great balance, neuromuscular coordination, speed, strength, and flexibility.

Soccer is unique because there are so many different demands. Just what factors of fitness seem to be important in soccer? (See the section on fitness testing later in this chapter for details on how best to test the fitness levels of soccer players.)

• *Aerobic capacity*: College/adult men typically run upward of 10,000 meters during a game, and elite women run slightly less. Of that 10,000 meters, about two-thirds of the total is covered at a walking or jogging pace. These low- or moderate-intensity speeds are fueled aerobically. In addition, soccer players run at higher intensities about once every 45 seconds and sprint about once every 90 seconds. In between, they have to recover for the next high-speed run. (Recovery is an aerobic activity that I will address in chapter 3.) Thus, in order to recover and run well the next time, a soccer player needs a good aerobic system. As good as that of a marathoner? Hardly. Actually, the endurance of a soccer player is fairly average when compared with that of other athletes. Typical vo_2 max (the maximum volume of oxygen used by the body) for a male soccer player is 55–65 milliliters/kilograms/minute, whereas that of a marathoner can be well into the 80s. The elite woman's results will be in the upper 40s to upper 50s.

• *Anaerobic capacity*: A 300-meter sprint is a good measure of anaerobic capacity, but when was the last time a soccer player had to sprint 300 meters? Anaerobic capacity is not a very important factor in soccer, a game that requires mostly moderate-intensity activity (walking/jogging), with short-duration, high-intensity running (10–40 meter sprints).

- *Strength*: This is usually measured as the weight one can lift once, and it is then related to body weight to compare different athletes. In soccer, strength is needed to tackle and resist charges. In testing, soccer players are consistent with other athletes but, like most others, are well below the really strong athletes like American football players and weight lifters.
- *Local muscle endurance*: This factor is about the length of time you work certain muscles. Doing lots of sit-ups tests local muscle endurance of the abdominal muscles. Because the situation changes so rapidly (every 5–6 seconds) in soccer, individual muscles seldom need to perform for a long time. But if you have to run, rest briefly, then do it all over again, local endurance of the legs is important. Plus, soccer emphasizes core (abdominal) muscle strength and endurance.
- *Speed*: Soccer players don't need world-class speed. Pay close attention and you will see that the sprint technique of most soccer players is pretty poor—nothing like that of a sprinter in track. Besides, it is difficult to run at top speed and try to control a ball, so most players sprint at just below top speed so they can be in control when they reach the ball. One of the biggest changes in the game over the years has been the speed of play. (Some might ask whether the speed seen today is running speed or speed of thought and decision making.) Good speed for adult male players is 8.5+ meters/second at top speed, while great sprinters are moving at 10+ meters/second.
- *Power*: This is usually measured by a vertical jump, and soccer players will not be dusting the top of too many backboards. Still, they have to be able to outjump an opponent for a head ball, and sometimes that opponent can be reaching with his hands. Typically, the best headers on a team have the best vertical jump. If you don't have the "ups," you are not likely to be in the middle of the box for a corner kick. Good jumps are 24 inches or more, with the best jumpers hitting 30+ inches, but still less than the 40+ inches we hear about in basketball. Vertical jump is hard to compare because there are different ways to measure it. When I hear of someone with a serious vertical jump, like 40 inches or more, I wonder how it was measured.
- *Balance*: This is tough to measure during movement. When run-

ning, if you get bumped, but you keep running, is that a demonstration of balance or some aspect of agility? Static balance tests of soccer players show decent results, but not as good as those of skaters or gymnasts.

- *Agility*: You know who has "it" and who doesn't. Actually, when soccer players perform agility tests, they routinely score at about the 99th percentile. Are they more agile than a point guard in basketball? We don't know, as a direct comparison hasn't been made. Plus, we don't know to what degree agility can be trained, but numerous soccer coaches and personal trainers with far more experience than I say it can be. All I am saying is that I haven't seen any controlled studies that confirm just how much agility is trainable within a season.
- *Flexibility*: Watch gymnasts and divers to realize what flexibility means. Soccer players tend to have poorer flexibility than most athletes, especially around the thigh, hamstring, and ankle.

There are other factors like neuromuscular performance (skills), body composition, and so forth. The take-home point is that soccer is the game of the masses, and no particular fitness traits are needed to play the game. Most trained soccer players have fairly average fitness test results when compared with other athletes—good in all aspects but not great in any one factor. However, agility is a factor in which soccer players seem to score very high.

ENERGY: THE CURRENCY OF EXERCISE

The toughest thing for most coaches to understand is the science behind sport. When it comes to training, that means the generation of energy for physical labor, which means biochemistry.

At its most basic element, exercise physiology comes down to two basic concepts: the ability of the body to *deliver* oxygen to the working muscles and the ability of the muscle to *use* the delivered oxygen. All the other factors of physiology simply support the delivery and use of oxygen. I personally think most coaching books go too far into physiology and biochemistry when explaining how the body responds to exercise and adapts to training. I'll be gentle.

The Delivery of Oxygen

For oxygen to be delivered somewhere, it has to have a way of being carried. Oxygen is carried by hemoglobin in red blood cells. Of course, there are many details regarding how oxygen is carried by the cells, but just understand that a red cell has only so much space to carry oxygen, and the blood can only have so many red cells before it becomes too thick. If you want to carry more oxygen, you need more red cells, thus the attempts at what is called "blood doping," where the blood, with its red cells, is removed, stored, and then reinserted to increase oxygen carrying capacity. The hard-core endurance athletes — cyclists and cross-country skiers, for example — experiment with blood doping. To my knowledge, no one has attempted blood doping in soccer. The other way to increase the blood's carrying capacity is to use drugs that simulate the hormone that produces red cells (erythropoietin, nicknamed EPO); if you've watched the big-time bike races, you've heard of EPO. Anyway, the point is that the blood will only hold so much oxygen, so there must be other ways to move more oxygen to the working muscles.

The heart is one remarkable organ. It works hard for a fraction of a second when it beats and then only needs fractions of a second to rest up for the next beat. And this goes on whether the heart rate is 60 or 200 beats per minute.

Let's start at rest. When at rest, the body is operating on what might be analogous to a car's idle — the minimum needed to operate. There is a certain energy requirement needed to keep things operating at idle, and this energy requirement is met mostly through energy production using oxygen. With a set content of oxygen in the blood, the heart pumps at a nice steady rate, sending all the oxygen needed to the body.

During exercise, the muscles must produce more energy, and they want to do this using oxygen. Now the body has two options. First, the muscles could just take more oxygen out of the blood that is going into the tissues. Muscle doesn't take all the oxygen out of the blood, so there is oxygen still there for the taking; blood never gets sucked dry of oxygen. The other option is for the muscles to take about the same amount of oxygen out of the blood but for the body to also pass more blood into the tissues.

Increased blood flow is brought about by increasing both the heart rate and the amount of blood pumped with each beat of the heart, called the stroke volume. The product of these two is a critical feature of exercise called the "cardiac output." During exercise, both heart rate and stroke volume increase up to a point. Stroke volume increases to about 40% of a person's capacity, then plateaus. Thus, in order to further increase the cardiac output, the heart rate must continue to increase.

The cardiovascular system responds to training in a number of ways. Probably the most obvious is related to heart rate. As a result of training, the resting heart rate is reduced, as is the heart rate at the same workload. If your heart rate before training for a 10 minute per mile jog is 170, it might be 150 at that same pace after training. Maximal heart rate is marginally affected and may actually drop by a few beats.

Stroke volume at rest rises due to the training effect. Oxygen use by the body at rest is relatively constant, and cardiac output is closely related to the oxygen requirement. After training, when you sit at rest the oxygen need is similar to that before training. This means the cardiac output is similar at rest before and after training. If the heart rate decreases with training, then the stroke volume must increase to keep the resting cardiac output constant. During exercise after training, the same stroke volume response occurs, just at a higher level. So, if the maximum heart rate is about the same after training, the bigger stroke volume is the adaptation that drives the increased cardiac output and eventually an increased amount of oxygen being delivered to the muscles.

The Use of Oxygen

Once oxygen is delivered by the cardiovascular system to the muscles, the muscles have to make good use of the delivered oxygen. Oxygen moves from one place to another by the process of diffusion—this is the downhill movement from a place of high oxygen concentration (blood) to a play of low oxygen concentration (cells, muscle in this case).

Remember, oxygen is carried by hemoglobin in the red blood cells. When blood enters the low oxygen environment of muscle, oxygen leaves the hemoglobin, passes into the blood, through the capillary vessel wall, through the muscle cell wall, and then into the muscle interior to a hemoglobin-like molecule called myoglobin. From myoglobin, the oxygen moves to the real engines of the cell, called the mitochondria, where the energy is actually produced.

"Making Energy"

I put this in quotation marks because we really don't make energy. Our energy comes from the sun; all we do is transfer energy, through the food we eat, from the sun to our bodies, where it becomes available for biologic work. The body is very bright. Unlike a car that has one fuel and one way to use that fuel, the body has multiple fuels and different ways to use them. In the body, energy is located in a molecule called ATP (adenosine triphosphate). The adenosine molecule has three phosphates attached to it. Most people think the phosphates are the energy, but the energy is in the "glue" that holds the phosphates to each other and to the adenosine. We get energy for cellular work when a phosphate splits off the ATP (three phosphates), releasing the energy and leaving an ADP (adenosine diphosphate, two phosphates). If needed, we can get energy from the ADP by splitting off a second phosphate, liberating the energy and leaving an adenosine monophosphate (AMP). It is estimated that if one could put all of the body's ATP in one place, it might fill up a glass somewhere between the size of shot glass and a small juice glass. So when ATP is used, we had better make more because we can run out really fast.

Unfortunately, the body isn't a perfect machine. Only about 40% of the energy released when ATP splits is used by the cell; the rest is released as heat. Ever wonder where your body temperature comes from? It's the result of the breakdown of ATP at rest, where 60% of the available energy is released as heat. It doesn't take much insight to see that during exercise more energy is needed (so more ATP is broken down); consequently, more heat is produced, and the body temperature rises.

Anaerobic Energy

The methods of energy production fall under one of two headings: aerobic and anaerobic. "Anaerobic" means in the absence ("an-") of oxygen ("aerobic").

ATP-PC system. This is the quickest, but most limited, way to get energy. The body is in a constant state of exchange of phosphates between molecules. Remember, ATP is the molecule where energy is stored between phosphate molecules. ATP isn't the only compound where energy is stored. Phosphate, and the subsequent energy, is stored when connected to creatine (yes, that creatine). When the energy in an ATP molecule is used, a phosphocreatine (PC) molecule transfers its energy and phosphate to the ADP. What is left is an ATP and a creatine. Soon, energy and a phosphate must be put back on that creatine so that PC can feed the next ADP. Now, if things get really tight for energy, the body will take two ADPs and transfer energy and a phosphate to one of the ADPs. Now an ATP and an AMP (which may end up as ammonia) are left. The body is continually transferring energy and phosphates around.

The lactate system. The body has a second anaerobic method of energy production. The starting point here is sugar—blood glucose or the storage form of glucose, glycogen. The chemistry of this process is difficult for most people, so I will try to simplify it.

The glucose molecule contains six carbons. This lactate system process breaks down glucose into two, three-carbon molecules and two new ATP molecules. At the end is a waste product called lactic acid. Don't worry about the chemistry of this process. Just accept it on faith.

This method of energy production is not as fast as making energy through the ATP-PC system, but it can make energy for a longer period of time. The problem is the waste product, which can upset the chemistry (the pH) of the muscle. So the body better have a way to make energy that doesn't potentially damage the tissue with low pH. Once lactic acid is produced, the body must work to get rid of it.

Aerobic System

The body is pretty well put together. When getting energy from glucose, in the absence of sufficient oxygen, the glucose remnants end up as lactic acid. With plenty of oxygen present, however, the glucose remnants go through a complex cycle of events and produce two basic products: carbon dioxide and a series of products that move to a short chain of events that transfer electrons (hydrogen ions) down the line. As these electrons are passed down the line, enough energy is accumulated to attach a phosphate to an ADP to make an ATP. Either two or three ATPs are produced, and the final stop in this process is where oxygen is used: to join with the hydrogens to form water (H_2O). I refuse to get into ATP counting—just accept it on faith that the metabolism of a glucose molecule yields thirty-six or thirty-seven ATPS, depending on where the process starts. This process is limited only by the amount of glucose available.

Remember, the body is not a car. We have multiple fuel sources, and we can also get energy from metabolizing fats. Some will say this is more complicated simply because fats give us way more ATP than does glucose. Just realize that fat is a much bigger molecule than glucose, and lots of pieces of a fat molecule go through aerobic energy metabolism—so many that a fat molecule can lead to over 200 ATPS, depending on the size of the fat molecule. Even the skinniest marathon runner has plenty of fat to supply energy for multiple back-to-back marathons. For all intents and purposes, to the exercising athlete fat is an inexhaustible supply of energy.

Finally, we can get some ATP from metabolizing proteins. However, proteins don't become a real factor until the stores of glycogen are about gone, and even then it may supply, at best, 15% of the energy during exercise.

ENERGY AND EXERCISE

Assuming you have grasped the concept of energy production, the next step is to understand how this all works together during exercise. One way to do this is to compare the capacity and rate of production for each method (table 2.1). Now, the intensity of an activity dictates the predominant source of energy. For a sprint, like a 20-yard sprint in soccer, you need energy for a 3-second burst. You need energy very fast but for a short period of time, so most (but not all) of the energy comes from the ATP-PC system. Now, imagine that the wing defender has made a long attacking run, but a teammate loses the ball, and now the defender has to track all the way back to his goal. This run is longer but at a slower pace than that 20-yard sprint. So he needs energy for a bit longer and can afford to get it at a slower rate. In this case, the lactic acid system is the predominant (but not the only) source of energy, with all the consequences of lactic acid production—that pain you feel in your legs after a run like this. At least this pain and fatigue are transient. Finally, when players are simply positioning and repo-

Method of Energy Production	Rate of Energy Production	Capacity to Produce Energy	TABLE 2.1
ATP-PC	Fastest	Very limited	Methods of Energy Production by Rate and Capacity
Lactic acid	Fast	Somewhat limited	
Aerobic	Slow	Virtually unlimited	

sitioning as the ball moves around the field, they move at a walk or a jog, meaning the rate of energy use is low, so the predominant supply system is the aerobic system, resulting in the easily eliminated waste products of water and carbon dioxide.

To repeat, the critical factor in determining what system is used is the intensity of the exercise. The faster that energy is needed, like for a shot, jump, tackle, or sprint, the more you rely on the ATP-PC system. For longer runs at a fast pace, you use the lactic acid system but pay a price with a painful waste product. For walking and jogging (remember, this is around two-thirds of the distance covered in a game), you can get energy at an almost leisurely rate when compared with the anaerobic methods.

Training

Remember, it's all about oxygen, delivering it and using it. Training aims to improve oxygen use first and foremost, to conserve the limited fuel source of muscle glycogen, and finally to increase the efficiency of oxygen use.

Improving oxygen use. This concept is pretty simple. Let's say that to run a 10-minute mile before training, you get 75% of the energy needed from the aerobic system and 25% of the energy from the lactic acid system. After a training program, go out and run that 10-minute mile again, and you may find that you get 90% of the energy from the aerobic system and 10% from the lactic acid system. Before training, the increased use of the lactic acid system means that lactic acid is produced. After training, the reduced reliance on this system means less lactic acid is produced, and the run feels easier. These effects are accomplished by both improved oxygen delivery and better oxygen use.

Conserving muscle glycogen. Let's stay with that 10-minute mile. In the lab we can determine how much of the energy comes from the metabolism of fats and how much comes from the metabolism of carbohydrates (glucose). So, before training, you run that 10-minute mile on the treadmill, and we may find out that you derived 75% of the energy from carbohydrates and 25% from fats. At this rate, you might run out of glycogen pretty soon. Most people start to run out of stored glycogen with 1.5–2 hours of exercise. After training, let's put you back on that treadmill at that 10-minute mile. We may see that this time you derived maybe 40% of the energy from carbohydrates and 60% from fats. Now, you are able to run at this pace for a longer time before running out of carbohydrate. And that's good.

Efficiency of oxygen use. The whole idea of training is to increase the intensity of exercise that can be fueled aerobically. During exercise, energy is derived aerobically and anaerobically from a mixture of carbohydrates and fats. As the intensity of exercise increases, more energy is derived anaerobically, but in doing so, lactic acid is produced. One way to look at the efficiency of oxygen use is to determine at what intensity of exercise is lactic acid produced faster than the body can get rid of it (meaning the acid spills out into the blood). In the untrained state, lactic acid might start spilling out into the blood at 65% of capacity. After training, we might see that lactic acid doesn't start to spill out into the blood until maybe 80% of capacity is reached. Now, if the 65% of capacity was jogging at an 8-minute mile pace, the 80% pace might now be a 6.5-minute mile—a good deal faster. When lactic acid builds up, you feel it and usually slow down. What does this mean in soccer? Simple. Your "jogging" pace, used to position yourself around the field, is faster than that of your untrained opponent. If your opponent tries to keep up, he or she will produce lactic acid and get tired, but you won't. When you have to run faster, you won't have the load of lactic acid screaming at you to slow down.

What else does the improved use of oxygen mean to the soccer player? Soccer is less about a great aerobic capacity and more about the ability to recover between runs, and recovery is an aerobic activity. To get rid of waste products, you continue to breathe hard to keep taking in oxygen, which eliminates wastes like lactic acid and also reestablishes PC levels. The better the aerobic system, the faster you recover, pure and simple. The whole idea is to teach the body that it will need to supply energy quickly and recover fast because you are going to be asking for lots of energy again and again and again. Which should be more important to the soccer player: being able to run 3 miles at a 6-minute pace or being able to run 50 yards in 6–7 seconds, only to do it again with 10 seconds of rest? You'd better say the latter.

The Individuality of Training

The typical commercial for soccer is that the game is 90 minutes of nonstop action. I have pointed out that, in reality, the ball is in play for more like 60–70 minutes because the various periods of time when the action is stopped, due to the ball being out of bounds, injuries, fouls, and so forth, add up. Then, I have also pointed out how far players run and that about two-thirds of that distance is covered at the lower intensities of walking and jogging; sprinting might cover a total distance of 800–1,000 meters (for adult males), mostly done in runs of 10–30 meters spaced 45–90 seconds apart. This means that aerobic fitness is critical for performance. In this section, I'll present some of the "academics" behind the logic of training and apply it all to soccer.

The most important factor that governs the response to training is genetics. Everyone responds to training in individual ways, even if the training performed by each player is identical. Some players respond better to endurance training, and others respond to shorter, more power/strength-based activities. Research has shown that genetics can account for between 25% and 50% of your endurance. One project put athletes through training programs and reported improvements in endurance of 0–43% after 12 months of training. All participants did the same thing, but they responded differently. The phrase is, "The best way to become an Olympic athlete is to be selective when choosing your parents."

Track and field is a good stage to look at sporting ability. The 100-meter sprinter has a very different makeup compared with the athlete who performs the 10,000-meter race. Sprinters are typically taller and more muscular. Their muscle cells (fibers) are predominantly fast-twitch muscle fibers (type II), whose characteristics are a fast contraction speed and a high power output. Type II fibers can be recruited for very high intensity exercise, and they generate energy anaerobically that can support short-term explosive activities such as sprinting. The muscle fiber characteristics of the 10,000-meter runner are just the opposite. The runner's muscles are mostly slow-twitch muscle fibers (type I). These muscle fibers contract slowly and generate low power output. They are associated with low-intensity exercise, generate energy aerobically, and are fatigue-resistant. Type I muscle fibers are best suited for moderate-intensity, long-duration exercise all the while resisting fatigue. Most muscles contain a mixture of the various muscle fiber types, and fiber distribution is different from one individual to the next. Each fiber type can be trained to a certain degree, but the relative composition of muscles is genetically determined. In the end, athletic and sporting capabilities are in large part genetically predetermined. One of the great things about soccer is that there are no genetic gifts necessary (like height in basketball) to play the game.

Initial fitness levels prior to training also govern one's response to training, especially for the injured and deconditioned athlete. After a period of inactivity, fitness levels are lower for these players compared with those who are still playing. Thus, if one starts training when out of shape or after an injury, the gains in fitness will be fairly rapid in comparison to the gains conditioned athletes get in their regular training—despite their higher fitness levels. The higher the starting point, the smaller the relative improvement from training. In other words, the more you have to gain, the more you gain.

Overload

In order to improve fitness, the training program must provide a sufficient stimulus, called "overload." It is really simple. To improve your fitness, you have to make the body work harder than what it is currently accustomed to, which will lead to adaptation and improved performance. A well-designed program of overload training will develop a reserve that the player can call on when needed. With a huge reserve, the game feels easier, fatigue is delayed, decisions are better, and overall performance is increased. The overload stimulus has to be progressive. If not, improvements will begin to level off, and performance will not continue to improve. For example, an athlete attempting to improve his bench press may start out with three sets of eight reps with a weight of 100 pounds on the bar. With many training sessions, the athlete's upper body strength will increase, the 100 pounds will feel lighter than when the training started, and the player will be able to perform more repetitions before fatigue. To continue to gain strength, the amount of weight used or the number of sets/repetitions performed will have to increase. Overload is applicable to virtually all forms of fitness training. Progressive overload is also a very important factor for injured and deconditioned athletes. The adaptation to retraining can be quick, but the overload must be continued in order to return the player to full competition. Failure to continue the overload results in less improvement in fitness, which leaves the player ill prepared to compete. So, how does one create an overload stimulus? By manipulating the primary factors of fitness: frequency, intensity, and duration of training.

Frequency, Intensity, and Duration of Training

No matter how you couch it, all training programs must contain the principles of frequency, intensity, and duration. Improvements in fitness will occur if any of these three factors are increased.

"Frequency" refers to the number of training sessions performed. There appears to be no magic number of days to train in order to bring about the optimal improvements for soccer. The frequency of sessions depends entirely on the goal of the training program or session. Is the goal of the program to improve endurance, strength, or power? Is the player training for a recreational league or some higher-level competition? While any added days of exercise will increase fitness, most people believe that three nonconsecutive training sessions a week is the minimum necessary to improve fitness (figure 2.1). It is also known that doing the same exercises every day can lead to overuse injury. To avoid overuse injuries, it is important to have rest days. Cross-training days need to be considered as a replacement for regular training. Some highly competitive teams train three times a day, but the goal of each session is usually different, so they aren't doing the same exercises in each session.

"Intensity" is usually thought of as a percentage of maximum capacity. The relationship between fitness improvement and exercise intensity is an S-shaped curve (figure 2.2). Small increases in intensity at the low (left) end of the curve lead to small increases in fitness, while the same relative increase in intensity at the moderate (middle) area of the curve leads to much larger increases in fitness. At the high-

FIGURE 2.1

Relationship between Training
Days per Week, Increase in Fitness,
and Rate of Injury

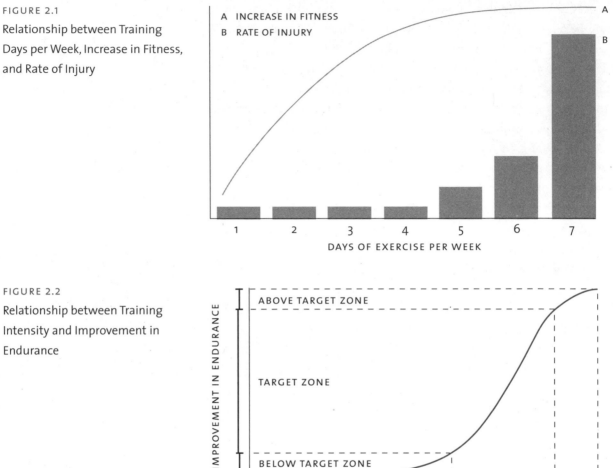

A   INCREASE IN FITNESS
B   RATE OF INJURY

DAYS OF EXERCISE PER WEEK

FIGURE 2.2

Relationship between Training
Intensity and Improvement in
Endurance

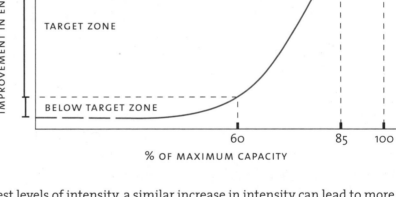

IMPROVEMENT IN ENDURANCE

ABOVE TARGET ZONE

TARGET ZONE

BELOW TARGET ZONE

% OF MAXIMUM CAPACITY

est levels of intensity, a similar increase in intensity can lead to more, but smaller, gains in fitness and are best left to the highly competitive elite athlete. Intensity can be measured on the field by heart rate or, more easily, by using a rating of perceived exertion.

"Duration" is the number of minutes spent at any particular intensity or the overall training session. Fitness levels increase up to about 45 minutes to 1 hour of work, and then further increases in duration lead to smaller changes (figure 2.3). As before, the extremes of duration are best left to the highly competitive athletes.

The product of the duration and frequency of training bouts is known as "volume." Volume can be increased either by increasing the

THE PERCEPTION OF EXERTION

0–10 Scale		6–20 Scale	
0	nothing at all	6	
.5	just noticeable	7	very, very light
1	very light	8	
2	light	9	very light
3	moderate	10	
4	somewhat hard	11	light
5	hard	12	
6		13	somewhat hard
7	very hard	14	
8		15	hard
9		16	
10	very, very hard	17	very hard
10+*	almost maximal	18	
		19	very, very hard
		20	

*Using the 0–10 scale, one can rate exercise intensity above a "10."

While some people use heart rate as a measure of exercise intensity, most people exercise to some perception of intensity. This latter method of measuring intensity is called the rating of perceived exertion (RPE). Use either of the following rating scales (the 0–10 or 6–20 scale) to answer this question: "How hard is the exercise?" The response is a number that corresponds to the appropriate keyword. For example, when estimating the RPE of jogging, most people will respond 3, 4, or 5 (or 12–15, using the 6–20 scale).

frequency or the duration of sessions. After all is said here, remember this: volume of training and intensity of training are inversely related. That means you can't train long *and* hard. It begs the obvious, but you wouldn't try to run a marathon at your 100-meter dash speed. This is due to the various energy systems employed to support energy production during short-, medium-, and long-term exercise at varying intensities. To do any work, you need to supply energy, and the body gets its energy two ways; anaerobic (in the absence of oxygen) and aerobic (in the presence of oxygen). Anaerobically, you get energy almost instantly, but the capacity (the total amount of available energy) is limited, meaning you don't work at very high intensities for very long because of fatigue that is in part related to waste products like lactic acid and ammonia. Aerobically, you get an unlimited supply of energy much more slowly and work of this magnitude produces

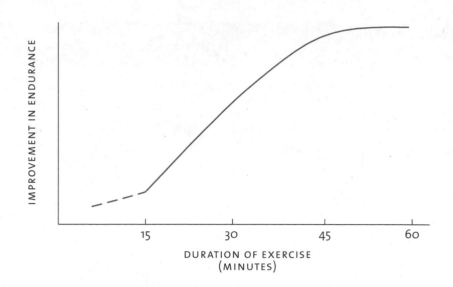

simple waste products like water and carbon dioxide, thus exercise can be maintained for extended periods of time.

Which of the three elements—intensity, frequency, or duration—will have the greatest effect on fitness levels? It appears that intensity is the critical factor. However, a structured training program should feature all three elements. Studies that have examined tapering (a reduction in training in order to peak for a particular event) show the importance of exercise intensity when attempting to maintain fitness levels. If you reduce training volume or frequency by 67% but maintain the intensity, fitness levels can be sustained for an astounding 15 weeks! As soon as intensity levels drop, though, fitness levels fall.

Specificity of Training and Cross-Training

The principle of specificity has a major role in the physiological responses to training, the body's adaptations that occur following training, and the mechanism of fatigue. Training should, as closely as possible, mirror the movement pattern and energy supply for the sport. While these concepts are discussed elsewhere in this book, they deserve repeating here.

Specificity of exercise. A specific exercise elicits a specific response. The heart rate of someone running a 100-meter sprint is a whole lot different than that of someone running 5,000 meters. In training for soccer, if you want the proper heart rate response, it is best to plan activities that mimic the game.

Specificity of training. A specific training program will lead to specific outcomes in the body. The adaptation of muscle to lifting weights is substantially different from the adaptation to a distance running program. Again, the best way to train for the game is to plan activities that are like the game. Distance running during the season will train a player to be a distance runner, not a soccer player.

Specificity of fatigue. The reason an athlete fatigues (fails to maintain a desired power output) when lifting weights is quite different from the reasons an athlete fatigues from distance running. Fatigue in soccer is from repeated short sprints, which deplete muscle glycogen, as well as dehydration.

Cross-Training

Despite the principle of specificity of training, athletes may improve their performance in one mode of training by training in another. Cross-training benefits the injured and deconditioned athlete by allowing participation in training even if the desired mode of training is not an option. For example, cycling enables an athlete to train aerobically, even if an injury prevents him from being able to run. He can thus maintain his cardiovascular fitness despite his injury. Numerous studies have reported that runners were able to maintain their running performances by running in deep water over a period of 4 weeks. With the correct volume and intensity, deep-water running offers aerobic benefits similar to those of actual running, which is why therapists use running in water when an athlete can't be on the field. Even the most serious athletes can get some benefits from cross-training, without increasing the risk of injury.

While cross-training can be effective, the bulk of the research arrives at the same conclusion: although cross-training may demonstrate some transfer effects of training, the size of the effects will be smaller than that which could be attained by increasing specific training by a similar amount. Still, if specific training is not possible, cross-training could be an option. Some training is better than no training. It appears that improvements in the cardiovascular system are more general. Anaerobic training is entirely specific, as these adaptations occur within the muscle. Muscles not used in training will not produce the desired response.

One February a few years ago, I spent a great weekend in Winchester, Virginia, where I spoke about knee injuries to physical therapy students at Shenandoah University and then had the opportunity to go watch a local girls' team train indoors under the steady eye of James Wood High School coach Dave Pennypacker. After watching an hour of training, Dave asked if I wanted to join in for scrimmage. "Oh, wait, let me think about it. . . . Sure." I agreed to play—three games to five. I learned something that night: Pain can be quite instructive.

I stepped on the floor with no warm-up, knowing better. I thought I would just take it easy, trap and pass and let the kids run. That lasted maybe 10 seconds. Within minutes, I was bent over, sucking wind harder than I could remember in recent history. I know what lactic acid buildup feels like, and I was way beyond buildup and was approaching overflowing. Would one of the girls *pleeeeease* score so we could take a break?

A score—finally—and I practically crawled to the water fountain. Okay, I know what I did wrong. No warm-up. I asked my body to go from standing and watching to short, high-intensity runs, dribbling, and trying to catch up to passes (doesn't anyone pass to feet anymore?). The low pH from the lactate buildup was making my legs feel so heavy and tired. Oh, no. Kickoff.

A little rest and water seemed to have done me good. The running was less stressful, the turns quicker, my ball control was improved, passes were crisper, and most important, ninth grade girls weren't making me look my actual age. I felt more like I knew (or remem-

bered) what I was doing. The fifth goal led to another break, but this break didn't feel like it really was needed. Let's get back to playing!

A few players were swapped, and off we went again. After a while some parents started showing up, the clue that we were about finish. I was tired, but I had had a good time. It wasn't long before I started to tighten up. I could hardly wait for the next day.

Saturday morning brought about more pain— and more learning. I hadn't been running much due to residual heel pain from an extended bout of plantar fasciitis, but I had been riding the stationary cycle, so my endurance was respectable. But my legs were *reeeeeeeally* sore. The front of my legs was sore because I hadn't used my ankles for all the needed foot positions. My calf muscles were sore because I hadn't sprinted in some time. My quads and hams were sore from running, from stopping, from kicking. But the most soreness was located in my adductor muscles—the groin muscles. You never know how much you use those muscles until they tell you with soreness the next day; it stems from all the pushing off when reaching for a tackle and changing direction.

The reason for the pain is pretty well understood. When muscles contract while lengthening, a great deal of force is generated and can damage muscle cell membranes. This result is an upset in the internal environment of the muscle, with damage to the part of the muscle that develops tension—the sarcomere—leading to pain the next day. Not much has been shown to prevent this soreness, although vitamins C and E seem to help speed up the repair.

This pain is evidence of damage, and it is one of the quickest adaptations by the body. An old coaching adage says to get rid of soreness, do again whatever it was that made you sore, and that is correct. Had I gone out and played the next day instead of watching TV, I wouldn't have felt nearly as bad on Monday as I did on Saturday. Play again, and the soreness would be even less.

So what value does the self-pity of an ex-player have for the current player or coach? How many times have you seen teams going through a fairly passive warm-up? A little ball work, some stretching, maybe a little 5v2, and it's time for kickoff. But the first 10–15 minutes of the game just don't seem to be clicking, though after a while things start to look better. The same thing can happen at the start of the second half. Why? The warm-up for the first half wasn't specific to the game—it was too passive, with not enough higher-intensity work prior to kickoff. And the second half? The players have just spent the last 15 minutes listening to a review of the first half and changes for the second half, and then are expected to step right out and play. Not good. Jens Bangsbo, the Danish researcher of soccer and once the first assistant coach for Juventus FC, has shown that the distance run during the start of the second half is low, probably because of the lack of warm-up.

What about the soreness? In order to be prepared for play, all players need to go through lots of changes of direction. Playing 11v11 in practice is not intense enough, not active enough—a theme I address over and over. Smaller-sided games require more of everything, so emphasis should be placed on these games. Straight-ahead running teaches a player to run straight ahead. Activities should require many changes of direction and agility work. Such training will make players better prepared for the quick changes of direction required in the game.

From a training theory standpoint, this is all called "specificity." The more specific the training is to the activity, the more appropriate the adaptations specific to the demands of competition will be. So don't send players out running straight ahead. Don't send them out to run high-intensity sprints in the game without having run some before the whistle. Specificity—a concept you are not allowed to ignore.

Reversibility of Training

If you don't train, due to illness, injury, or general laziness, a lot of the gains in fitness can be lost in as few as 10 days. This "detraining" happens regardless of one's preexisting state of physical fitness and has different effects on aerobic and anaerobic fitness. The loss of aerobic power is considerably greater than that for other performance capacities, such as strength, power, and flexibility. In a famous study in 1968, the effects of complete bed rest on fitness levels were studied. Five subjects were confined to bed for 20 straight days, and their aerobic capacity declined by 25% (approximately 1% per each day of rest!). This decrease was largely due to a reduction in cardiac performance, and these reductions occurred in the first 12 days of detraining. A clear illustration of the effect of detraining is highlighted in figure 2.4. Capillary density (the denser the capillary network, the less distance oxygen must travel to get to the muscle), aerobic enzymes, and ultimately VO_2 max all reflect the efficiency of a person's aerobic capacity. The graph shows that improved fitness levels that took almost 2 years to achieve were lost within only 6 months of detraining. Decreases in muscular endurance performance can occur very rapidly following the complete cessation of training because of the muscles' impaired ability to generate energy aerobically and anaerobically. Detraining can occur as quickly as 2 weeks if immobilization has occurred; however, if muscles are able to move freely, then a minimal amount of training stimulus should be sufficient to prevent substantial drops in muscular endurance.

Improvements lost during detraining are not regained at the same rate as fitness was lost. If an athlete stops training for 12 days, only 75% of the aerobic enzymes are regained after 24 days of retraining. As one study found, if you retrain for 15 days after having laid off training for 15 days, your aerobic enzymes and VO_2 max will not have returned to preexisting levels, and your endurance performance will be slower by two minutes.

Everyone, regardless of fitness level, demonstrates a slow return to fitness when compared with the rate of loss. This means that detraining is a fast process, and retraining is a slow process. This adds credence to that old coaching saying: "It's easier to stay in shape than it is to get in shape."

Maintenance of Fitness

This all begs a question: what can be done to maintain fitness? In other words, what is the least one can do to maintain fitness? Remember, training is a mixture of three factors: training frequency (days per week), training intensity, and training duration (minutes per day). All three have to be considered when figuring out how to maintain fitness.

- *Reduction in frequency*: If the number of training days is reduced by one-third or two-thirds (from 6 training days per week to 4 or 2 days per week) and the training intensity and duration are main-

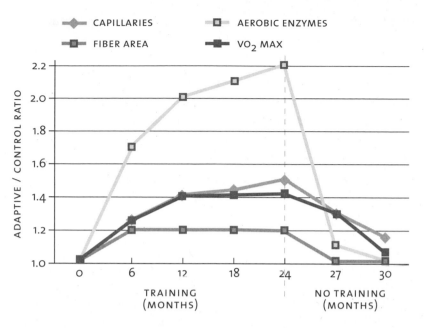

FIGURE 2.4

Physiological Responses
to Training and Detraining
Source: Adapted from B. Saltin et al.,
"Fiber Types and Metabolic Potentials
of Skeletal Muscles in Sedentary Man
and Endurance Runners," *Annals of
the New York Academy of Sciences*
301 (1977): 3–29.

tained (that is, one works as hard and as long as before), it is possible to maintain endurance.

• *Reduction in intensity*: If training intensity is reduced by one-third or two-thirds and the training frequency and duration are maintained (one works as frequently and as long), there are significant reductions in endurance.

• *Reduction in duration*: If the minutes per session are reduced by one-third or two-thirds (from 40 minutes per session to 26 or 13 minutes per session), but the training frequency and training intensity are maintained (one works as hard and as often), it is possible to maintain endurance.

This means that frequency and duration can be reduced with little effect on overall endurance *if* intensity is maintained. The quickest way to lose endurance is to reduce training intensity. It is important to keep practicing at a training intensity similar to what one achieves during the season. Following an injury, joints and their surrounding muscles may be immobilized. The detraining process in muscle occurs very, very rapidly. Anyone who has ever had an injury requiring a cast or other immobilizer has noticed muscle wasting (called atrophy or hypotrophy). Muscle size is reduced, which leads to reductions in muscular strength and power. Unlike aerobic capacity, reductions in neuromuscular performance are not as rapid following detraining. If muscles are not placed in a cast, large drops in strength can be minimized because the muscles can move around freely. The detraining process has a more pronounced effect on aerobic performance than it does on anaerobic performance (strength, power, and muscular endurance). The loss of endurance is primarily due to a reduction in the ability to generate aerobic energy. Strength, power, and muscular endurance can all be maintained to a certain degree via one high-intensity training session per week. However, maintaining aerobic capacity requires two days a week of training, if the intensity of the exercise is high (85–100% VO_2 max).

WARM-UP

The general purpose of warm-up is simple: to prepare the body for exercise. The properly warmed-up muscle seems to be more resistant to injury. The metabolic processes that make energy available function more effectively at temperatures slightly higher than body temperature. The warm muscle produces energy quicker and resists injury better than a "cold" muscle.

Warm-up can be either general or very specific. General warm-up activities include calisthenics, stretching, and general "loosening up" activities unrelated to the upcoming game. I even had an English player years ago who would take a warm shower or ask for a massage as a means of general warm-up. Specific warm-up includes performing the upcoming exercise at a reduced intensity.

The benefits of warm-up can be psychological, as well as physical. The mental preparation for a contest allows the athlete to get a "feel" for how he thinks he will perform. I used to do a lot of jumping during warm-up to let me know if I had the hops that day. Strikers shoot to see if their shot is "on" that day. To give the athlete confidence going into the match, the warm-up activities should be done accurately and precisely—do it poorly, and the player thinks, "Oh, no. My left foot is really off today."

The psychological side of warm-up may be a little difficult to prove, but the physical side of warm-up is well studied. Physiologically, warm-up helps the body in five ways:

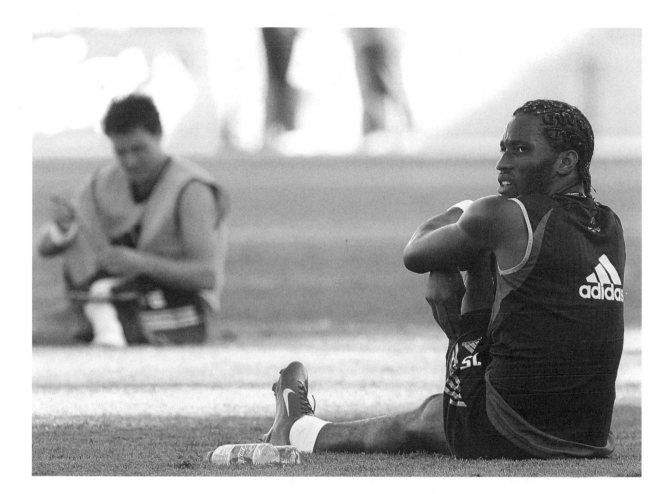

1 Speed of muscle function and relaxation is increased.
2 Movements by a warm muscle are more efficient.
3 Oxygen moves through warm muscles more quickly.
4 Nerve transmission and energy metabolism are improved.
5 There is increased blood flow through the warm muscles (obviously specific to the muscles warmed up).

Chelsea practice session before the 2006 Major League Soccer All Star Game. Stretching is known to protect against injury. Take your time and do a thorough job. (Photograph by Tony Quinn; SoccerStock.com)

Warm-up activities should begin as general activities to break a sweat and then move to the more specific exercises, with gradually increasing intensity. Don't do too much or go so hard so that fatigue sets in. A good all-purpose guideline is that once you have broken a sweat from the warm-up, the body is probably prepared to play. Fifteen to twenty minutes or more is not unusual for a warm-up. It is

Exercises for this routine were borrowed from places like the English FA, F-MARC, Santa Monica Sports Medicine, Vern Gambetta, Pierre Barrieu, and others. This routine proceeds after 5–10 minutes of general, light jogging. Adjust the number of reps or sets to suit your age group and level of fitness.

Activity	Elapsed Time
Jog, sideline to sideline	0–.5 minutes
Shuttle: Start one direction leading with right leg, stop at midfield, return leading off with left leg	.5–1 minute
Backward running, sideline to sideline	1–1.5 minutes
Calf stretching (30 seconds each leg): Two players on opposite sides of ball, with straight leg and heel on ground; put ball of foot on ball to stretch calf	1.5–2.5 minutes
Standing thigh stretch (30 seconds each leg): Stand on one leg, grab other ankle behind back, and stretch thigh; use partner for balance	2.5–3.5 minutes
Figure 4 hamstring stretch (30 seconds each leg): While seated, one leg is straight and other leg is bent, and foot touches knee of leg being stretched	3.5–4.5 minutes
Inner thigh stretch (30 seconds each leg): Seated, spread legs, lean forward trying to put chest on ground	4.5–5.5 minutes
Hip flexor stretch (30 seconds each leg): In forward lunge position, back knee on ground, lean forward stretching hip muscles	5.5–6.5 minutes
Walking lunges, 3 sets of 10 reps: Push off with right and lunge with left, drop right knee down; keep control, you should be able to see toes of lead leg	6.5–7.5 minutes
Russian hamstrings, 3 sets of 10 reps: Kneel on ground, partner holds ankles, keep back and hips straight, then lean forward, then back up straight (probably not for players with bad back)	7.5–8.5 minutes
Single toe raises, 30 reps each leg: On one leg, no support, slowly rise up on toes, slowly lower	8.5–9.5 minutes

Activity	Elapsed Time
Lateral hops over cones, 20 reps: Two-footed hops back and forth over cone 6 inches to your side	9.5–10 minutes
Forward and backward hops, 20 reps: As above, only forward and backward	10–10.5 minutes
Single leg hops over cones, 20 reps each leg: Forward and backward over cone; keep bend to knee; don't land on straight leg	10.5–11 minutes
Phantom headers, 20 reps: Pause between jumps, bend knees to take off and land; land on balls of feet	11–11.5 minutes
Scissors jumps, 20 reps: Forcefully push off with right leg, draw left leg up high, and land on ball of foot with bent knee; maintain control when landing	11.5–12 minutes
Shuttle run, forward and backward: Cruise or sprint between cones set about 10–20 yards apart	12–13 minutes
Diagonal runs: Fast run 10–15 yards, plant and cut about 45 degrees to right, then run and repeat to left; maintain control of knee of plant leg	13–14 minutes
Bounding run: Long strides with high knee lift; land on ball of foot and bent knee	14–15 minutes

best to start playing fairly soon after the warm-up because the benefits are quickly lost at rest.

When to stretch? A warm muscle responds better to stretching better than a cold muscle. So, perform a general warm-up, then stretch, then do a brief general warm-up, again followed by more extensive specific activities. The coaching adage is "warm-up to stretch, don't stretch to warm-up." In addition, warm-up should also include exercises designed for injury prevention. Finally, don't forget that a warm-up is needed for the second half. Far too many teams end up using the first 15 minutes of the second half as a warm-up because the coach has said way more than the players can absorb at halftime. If the other team has been warming up while your team was sitting, watch out: they will be all over your team because they are ready to play.

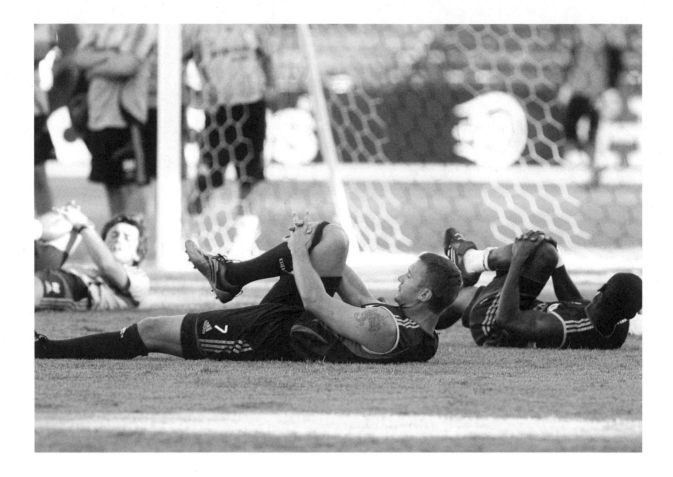

SPEED DEVELOPMENT FOR SOCCER

Chelsea practice session before the 2006 Major League Soccer All-Star Game. Stretch after your body is warmed up and again after training or a match. (Photograph by Tony Quinn; SoccerStock.com)

You may have already figured out that the fitness component that is most important to success is soccer-specific endurance: a good aerobic capacity to speed recovery from fast running. What I haven't addressed is the faster running part of that statement—speed. University of North Carolina men's coach Elmar Bolowich sees many teams that make little attempt to develop speed. I should be sensitive to the speed issue, too. Probably the main factor that got me a starting job when playing in college was that I was much faster than the competitor for my position, even though he was far better tactically than I. Most aspects of the game a coach can make accommodations for, but speed isn't one of them. It is hard to figure out how to counter a really fast team. All things being equal, the faster team will usually prevail.

In the mid-1950s the nature of the game was changed forever

when the great Hungarian national team destroyed, dismantled, and wholly embarrassed England 6-3 at Wembley—a game that was not as close as the score indicated. Observers of that game commented on the remarkable speed and work rate of the Hungarians. The Hungarians had four or five players who could run 100 meters in 11.5 seconds or less! I first started paying really serious attention to the World Cup in 1974 and read that all the field players from the former East Germany could run 100 meters under 11 seconds—from four to five players under 11.5 seconds to the *entire team* under 11. Nowadays, 11.5-second speed might not be fast enough for a good high school team.

The game I see today is played so much faster than the game I played. Is that a result of better athletes, better coaching, or something else? I would like to think it is the first two, but I also see coaches using the free substitution rule to encourage players to run as fast as they can—get tired and then be pulled for a rest. So players have the mindset to sprint whenever they are on the field. Recent National Collegiate Athletic Association (NCAA) men's finals have seen teams that try to play at a high pace for the entire game face teams that play at a more controlled pace and use speed selectively, like past winners Wisconsin, St. John's, and University of North Carolina.

Speed is an elusive creature. Is it innate, or can it be developed? What goes into the concept of speed? The first player to the ball may not be faster than the opponent; some people just consistently get there first. The great Larry Bird of the Boston Celtics was never to be confused with a sprinter, but he always seemed to be in the right place. Was it speed afoot or speed of thought, or both? Ajax Amsterdam uses its TIPS plan to evaluate 16-year-olds—in technique, intelligence, personality, and speed—and it considers speed the trait with the least potential for improvement.

The University of Pittsburgh coach, Joe Luxbacher, describes speed as having seven components: *perceptual speed* (using the senses to decipher various elements of game); *anticipation speed* (predicting what will happen before it happens); *decision-making speed* (making decisions in the shortest amount of time); *reaction speed* (reacting to some action by a teammate or opponent); *speed without the ball* (maximum movement speed); *speed with the ball* (movement with the ball at highest possible speed); and *game action speed* (making effective tactical decisions to changing conditions).

If you look closely at this list, you will see that many of the different aspects of speed are related to speed of thought and decision making. These are skills that can only be developed by playing the game. Yes, "the game is the best teacher"; however, you can help it a bit. It is fairly easy to modify small-sided games to require players to recognize, anticipate, decide, react, and act more quickly. Just reducing the size of the field puts more players in a smaller space, so defenders are on the attacker quicker. This forces both offense and defense to speed up the thought process. A half-field game of six on six can be speeded up dramatically by playing in the penalty area. Obviously, players need very good skills to be successful (the "T" of the Ajax TIPS program). In such games, the opponent grabs a missed trap very easily. Players who don't have good skills cannot play in a game like this. Many defensive tactics used today are in fact geared toward reducing the size of the field and putting more players in a smaller space.

Physically, the development of speed is largely based on improvement in running form. From experience I can say that the running form of soccer players will never be confused with that of a sprinter in track. In addition, remember that agility and speed are two different animals. The fastest players are not necessarily the most agile, and the most agile may not be the fastest. Elements of agility and lateral speed involve recognition, reaction, decisions, balance, footwork, change of direction, and avoiding obstacles.

Straight-Ahead Speed
Speed is part mental (decisions and anticipation) and part mechanical (running technique). Straight-ahead speed has been broken down by conditioning specialists like Vern Gambetta as starting speed, acceleration, top speed, deceleration, and cooperative speed (think of the running back who outruns his blocking).

Starting speed is largely a response to some stimulus and involves a series of cognitive processes. Consider a defender covering a striker. The striker's midfielder sees the striker open, looks down, and strikes the ball. Who gets to the ball first? In order to intercept that pass, a number of decisions must be made quickly by the defender: what space is the striker moving to? Is the ball played to feet or space? How is the ball moving? What is your speed? What is your opponent's speed? (That was the first thing I tried to judge when competing.)

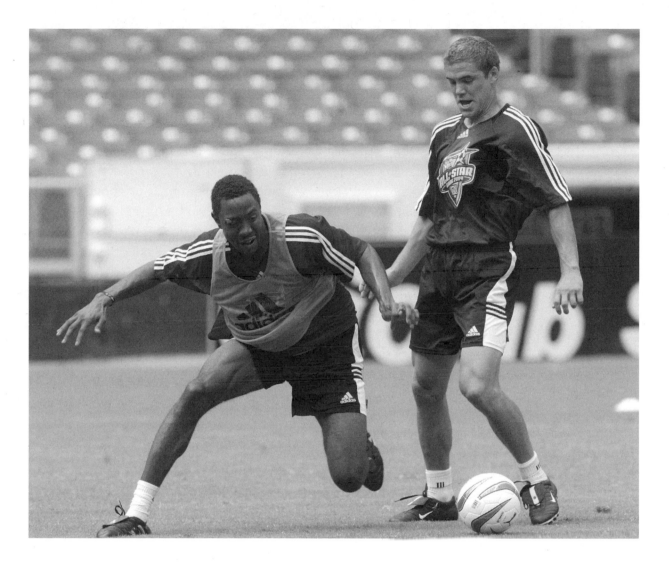

When should you start running to beat your opponent to the ball? How about the pace and spin on the pass? How do you time your response to the pass in relation to the striker's speed? Is the ball on the ground or in the air? If it's in the air, you must plot out the flight of the ball and determine where on the field and on your body (head, chest, foot, etc.) to first contact the ball, then add in the opponent's skills and speed. Then factor in what to do with the ball once you get it. Control? Head the ball? One-touch? Two-touch? Shot? Clear? To whom/where? All of this and more has to be considered in fractions of a second, every time something changes with the ball. This kind of thought process is the real playing of soccer. You've got to think fast

Practice session before the 2004 Major League Soccer All-Star Game. Changing directions can be hard on the knees. Keep the hip, knee, and foot aligned to protect the knee against injury. (Photograph by Tony Quinn; SoccerStock.com)

to play this game. These are all part of those mental features of the game that end up testing a player's speed of thought and reactions. These decisions aren't reflexes; these are reactions—not the same thing. A reflex, like the knee-jerk reflex, doesn't involve the brain. A reaction does require the brain; a player has to process and interpret input from many sources and then decide on a coordinated response.

How does one get better at this aspect of the game? Deliberate practice and repetition. Some say the real difference between the elite and the lower levels is that the elite player has practiced his or her skills so much that the execution of the skills is second nature; they are performed on a subconscious level, so to speak, that lets the conscious part of the brain focus on tactics, not the skills themselves.

The running part of speed also can be improved. This, too, is a mental project because improvement in running speed is largely the result of changing how one runs, refining the skill. In soccer, improvement in top-end sprint speed is not all that important. Why? Look at 100-meter sprinters. These runners don't reach top speed until the middle third of the race; it takes 30 meters to reach top speed. In soccer, full, all-out sprints (i.e., over 30 meters) are pretty rare. Most runs are of 30 meters or less.

What that means is that the time spent teaching one to increase top-end sprint speed might be time better spent on other lessons—like how to approach the first 30 meters of a run, where the player is reacting and accelerating, but never quite reaching top speed. Thus, the initial steps are important.

Speed expert and pro trainer Vern Gambetta taught me nearly everything I know about speed, so pay attention to his teachings. He breaks the form for the first steps down and names three factors as critical: posture, arm action, and leg action.

- *Posture*: Most people bend at the waist when running, especially when taking off. While it is correct to lean forward when accelerating, the lean should actually stem from the ankle, not the waist.
- *Arm action*: We all know the arms and legs work together diagonally—right leg and left arm forward. An exaggerated arm action in height and rate of arm swing helps the leg action when running fast.

- *Leg action*: In the first four to six steps the player should focus on pushing against the ground in such a way as to propel the body forward. This is where many young players err. They mistakenly think that by taking big first steps, they will cover a lot of ground fast. If that first step is long, then they are actually slowing themselves down by applying a braking force until their body gets over and beyond this lead foot and they can start pushing against the ground to go forward. If these first few steps are short, all their effort goes into pushing against the ground and propelling themselves forward. After four or five steps, they can stand more erect and bring their hips under their trunk.

Warming Up for Speed Training

It is very important to prepare the muscles for speed work. This kind of high-intensity work can cause an unprepared muscle to pull (strain). Warm-up seems to protect muscles from strains. Popular activities include pendulum swings of the legs both sideways and front to back, carioca with long strides, short strides, in a partial squat, and standing tall, high-stepping, high and long reaching, "volley traps," and passive stretches of the hamstrings, quads, and groin. Some people like using hurdles and elastic bands.

Teaching Acceleration

The following is Gambetta's progression for teaching acceleration:

- *Posture*: Start in the time-honored "ready position," with the legs bent, feet shoulder-width or more apart, and arms loose at the sides. Girls really need to learn this position. For some reason, they don't get into this position properly. Now, lean and take five short (and quiet) steps forward walking; turn and repeat the sequence jogging, stressing short steps. Next, with a partner facing in front, the player leans straight forward, and the partner uses his hands to catch the player by the shoulders. The player should keep his body straight and hold the position for about 5 seconds, getting used to the feeling of leaning at the ankles, not the hips. Now, repeat the exercise by running out eight to ten steps, emphasizing the first four to five, which should be short strides. Finally, repeat without the partner—lean forward at the ankle into short strides for eight to ten running steps.

- *Arm action*: Arm action can be practiced while stationary, though some players might think it looks odd to spectators. Standing, perform a very exaggerated arm swing, as though you were running, all the way up, down, and way back. Then sit straight-legged and repeat, only now the arms are bent so as to not hit the ground. Do a lot of these. With vigorous arm swinging while seated, the player can almost raise her seat off the ground. Now stand, feet staggered, with the right hand up in front of the face and the left back at the hip. On command, switch arm positions as fast as possible. Repeat this process lots of times, switching then stopping each time.

- *Leg action*: Leg action is trained with a partner, too. First, do some knee hugs by bringing the bent leg and knee as close to the chest as possible—hug it in. Next, repeat that partner drill where the player leaned into the partner and the partner caught the shoulders. Only this time, the partner resists while the player pushes for four to six strides. Then, vary this with the partner resisting strong for three to four steps, loosening up for three to four steps, then quickly letting go, turning, and running off so that the player must chase. Finally, the player leans into the partner and hugs a knee. The partner releases, and the player now must get the foot down and take off to run out.

Other activities for acceleration can help a player get used to feeling the speed. For example:

- If there is a slight slope, do these drills going downhill, or do the takeoffs downhill.
- Walk, then on command, execute these new skills to accelerate into a run.
- Do two-legged hops forward or to the side, then on command sprint out as fast as possible.
- Do a carioca then sprint out in any direction.
- Jump back and forth over a line or soft obstacle (cone, gym bag, etc.) three to five times, then sprint out.
- Scramble up from a push-up position and sprint out.
- Take the first step in one direction and move off in another direction.

• Do a two-footed jump, then on landing do a 180 and take off, all the while using the proper forms of posture, arm action, and leg action.

Lateral Speed and Agility

Watch any game and you will see some players who can cover distances very fast and others who seem to be able to navigate congestion in the penalty area with ease. The player who is accomplished at both is rare. Numerous research reports show that agility and speed are two completely different skills.

Pittsburgh's Luxbacher says that agility, like speed, has many components. These include *recognition/reaction* (recognizing the situation and reacting as soon as possible), *decision-making speed* (moving as fast as possible while assessing game situations), *balance/body awareness* (controlling and knowing where all body parts are all the time), *footwork* (having full control of the feet), *change of direction* (rapidly and accurately changing direction), and *obstacle avoidance* (reacting quickly to obstructions in the running path). Improving agility improves quickness both on and off the ball and body control, and it prevents injury.

Footwork is critical to agility. A common error is a short back step before moving in the desired direction, which lengthens the total reaction time. The more proper "first steps" are the crossover step (used for great distances—the back foot crosses over the front foot while the main push is from that front foot), open step (the lead foot steps out—not too far—and the push comes from the back foot), jab step (the lead foot steps slightly back and turns in desired direction—the push comes from the back foot), and the drop step (the lead foot drops straight or diagonally back while the push comes from the back foot). I could never do the drop step—a European teammate in college said I had "American feet." Picture this: You are facing the dribbler who manages to give a feint to your right and go around you to your left. My European friend would take the feint. Now his right foot is out where he took the feint and the left foot is back; basically the starting position of the drop step. Instead of running around this foot placement (like me), he would just swivel left on his feet (no steps) as they were planted and end up with the ball at his feet. Try it. It works. Quickly recognize the situation, drop step, turn, and there is the ball.

My friend could do this so quickly he would get called for obstruction (by American refs who didn't understand the move) and then get very mad. Our college once played a seriously good English team while we were touring England, years before such tours became commonplace. One of the many skills the English players demonstrated in their destruction of us was the ability to cut in one step what took us three to four steps to do.

So what kinds of activities improve agility? Try some of these:

1 A partner holds a ball in each hand and faces another player. The partner drops both balls, and the player must control both balls before the second bounce.

2 Shadow runs: A player in front runs the field with another player shadowing every move. Encourage the front player to change speed and direction often, with quick and rapid changes and accelerations. Also do this exercise with both facing each other so that the shadow player does the opposite of his partner.

3 Jumping rope is great. Try some of these variations: typical two-foot jump, stride jumps (swap the forward foot on each jump), crossover jumps, single-leg jumps.

4 Line steps: Stand to the side of a field line or rope, step over the line with the near foot and then the trail leg as fast as possible, then back. See how many can be done in 10 seconds. To make it harder, do this over a cone, balled-up towel, or other barrier. Don't use a ball as there is a danger of stepping on the ball, leading to a fall or a sprained ankle or worse.

5 A speed ladder is a vinyl "ladder" you roll out on the field. Run through (always as fast as possible) with one foot in each space. Then do two-foot jumps forward. Then try standing sideways on the left and stepping the right foot in, then the left foot in, then out to the right, then back to the left, and so on. Also try lateral crossover steps. Shuffle sideways straight through the ladder leading with the left foot, then back leading with the right. Some ladders have different distances from rung to rung, and that is fine. A speed ladder is a good investment. It is priced so that virtually any team can afford one or two.

6 In the "ready position" and on command, hop and turn 90 degrees, plant, then immediately return back to the front. On the

next command, turn in the other direction. Football players do this exercise a lot. It's very effective.

7 Set up corner flags in a slalom course (not always in a straight line). Players run fast through the course, emphasizing the plant of the outside foot, and cut tight around the flag. Girls, who are particularly susceptible to knee injury, should run this low, bending at the hips and knees. To emphasize body control, do this in flats, not studded soccer shoes.

8 5-10-5 shuttle: Going sideways, each player runs as fast as possible 5 yards to the right, 10 yards to the left, then 5 back to the right.

9 Icky Shuffle: Use the speed ladder and stand to the left to start. Always lead with foot next to the ladder. Step in with the right, follow with the left, then out to the right with the right foot, then into the next space with the left, follow with the right, then out with the left, etc. It looks like the Icky Shuffle, for those of you old enough to remember that. Try this going backwards, too.

10 Still using the speed ladder, hop to one foot landing in the space, hopping to two feet out, then back in landing on the other foot and so on.

11 Back to number 6. Now do the jumps turning 90 degrees and back to the front, then 180 degrees and back, then 270 degrees, and finally 360 degrees. Do this in both directions.

There are literally hundreds of drills one can do to improve agility. Basketball and football coaches are good resources, as are numerous books on conditioning. Check your local library or bookstore—especially for anything written by Vern Gambetta.

PRINCIPLES OF RECOVERY

While it should be obvious, sometimes it requires saying: changes in the body in response to training occur only during periods of rest. Training is all about balancing quality work and quality rest. It does little good to perform great training sessions without sufficient rest between sessions. In the absence of rest periods, hard session after hard session will soon become counterproductive. This also applies to competition. With players on multiple teams playing in league

Q How often should speed training be done?

A For high school or college players, some of these activities should be done 4 days a week: 2 days, a day off, then 2 more days. Club teams that only meet twice a week should do a little of each when training, but players should be encouraged to do some on their own two more times a week.

Q You mean do speed/acceleration and lateral speed/agility exercises at each workout?

A You probably should plan on 2 days for each, say Monday and Thursday for speed/acceleration and Tuesday and Friday for lateral speed/agility. If the team practices only twice a week, then insert a little of each during training.

Q Is there a preferred time in a practice?

A As these activities teach technique and footwork, training should be early in practice. A fatigued player will not be able to be to perform the skills properly.

Q Should speed training be done all year?

A Probably not. Early off-season training is usually low intensity and high volume. So speed training should begin closer to arrival to preseason training and during the season.

Q How many exercises?

A Variety is a good idea, so select 4–8 drills per practice and rotate activities each session.

Q Should everybody do these?

A Absolutely. Don't pigeonhole players according to position. Position-specific physical training is for the elite.

Q These are short-length activities. What should the work to rest ratio be, and what should be done during recovery?

A This training is for running technique, not "fitness" per se. So allow recovery to occur. A ratio of 1 to 3 should be the minimum, with full recovery the goal. Speed training is not used to improve endurance via interval training. During recovery, the players can stretch or do individual ball skills. Standing around only leads to mischief, as coaches well know.

Q Can a few days or weeks be taken off?

A Not a good idea. Repetition is important. There is a training concept called reversibility—more commonly called "use it or lose it."

Q At what age should training like this be added?

A Probably around middle school. Younger players need time to work on ball skills more than this.

Q Any suggestions for game day?

A Warm-up for competition should prepare the athlete for what is coming, which includes some high-speed running. A series of 5–6 short sprints in the final 5 minutes or so before kickoff is advised.

Some comments to keep in mind:

- Train when rested so proper technique is learned.
- Demand correct mechanics. The Lombardi quip is the goal: practice doesn't make perfect; perfect practice makes perfect.
- Top speed is not the goal. The optimum speed that one can control is the goal; changes in speed or

direction should be executed without having to "run around" the cut.

- Improvement in speed requires both motivation and concentration.
- A takeoff begins with a controlled fall (lean at the ankles), not leading with the head and shoulders (don't bend at the waist).
- Don't forget the arms. Arms initiate the movement. The bigger the arm swing, the more force applied to the ground.
- Short first steps get up to speed faster, much faster than big first steps.
- Extend at the ankle, the knees, and the hips for the best push against the ground.

- To slow down, absorb shock by the hips, knees, and ankles. Do not try to stop with one step. Lowering the body absorbs shock better with less risk of injury.
- Once these skills have been practiced, they must be applied at game speed. So plan activities for later in the practice that will force game-related speed for players to have a chance to implement these new skills at speed.
- Stress anticipation of actions so that players can learn to react faster to either the ball or other players.

games, tournaments, and other competitions, the only time some players get any quality rest is when they are injured. On the other hand, too much recovery will not help to boost fitness levels because infrequent training will not provide sufficient overload.

Remember the principle of overload; training must be at a workload above what the body is already accustomed to. Adaptation to training means that muscles and energy systems undergo physiological and structural improvements, permitting them to reset to a higher level. Recovery means the repletion of energy, repair of structural tissue damage, and recovery for the nervous system (which tends to take longer to recover than muscles). If the central nervous system is still fatigued during subsequent training bouts, nerve cells will fire at a slower rate, the number of muscle fibers recruited will be fewer, and movements will become less coordinated.

The rate at which energy stores are replenished following exercise depends on (1) the training intensity and (2) the energy systems utilized for that training session. Both of these factors go hand in hand. Muscle ATP and PC stores are returned to normal within a matter of minutes; however, carbohydrate stores can take up to 2 days to return to their pre-exercise level following exhaustive endurance exercise (distance running), which soccer is not. Muscle glycogen stores after intermittent running can be restored within 24 hours. The rate at which muscle glycogen stores are resynthesized largely depends on the timing and quality of carbohydrate intake after the workout or match. Carbohydrate intake should start right after exercise because the activity of the enzymes that lay down new glycogen is greatest in the first 2 hours right after exercise. A high carbohydrate diet will replenish muscle glycogen stores within 24 hours of exhaustive exercise, and most workouts are not exhaustive.

Training causes a certain amount of muscle damage, too. This damage is quickly repaired in preparation for the next training bout. If another training session is performed before the muscles have had the chance to repair, then you have the problem of insufficient rest. Thankfully, selected aspects of muscle repair are among the fastest adaptations to training. Studies have shown that after exercise the muscle protein repair (resynthesis) rate increases by 50% 4 hours after exercise and can climb to an 109% increase after 24 hours, then returns to baseline 36 hours after heavy training. Thus, it takes a period of up to 36 hours for recovery within muscles to be complete, and it is important that this period of recovery not be interrupted by another bout of training unless a prolonged rest period is planned (like a weekend of rest). However, you don't have to wait 36 hours in between every training session. The recovery process will be specific (there is that word again) to the nature of the prior training. Some professional athletes train up to three times a day, but each session has a different objective. Regardless of the objective of the training session, the wise coach will allow at least 6 hours between training sessions, as some indicators of training stress have returned to normal by this time.

Following a strenuous resistance or aerobic training session, muscle soreness is common. You can feel sore immediately after exercise, which can last for a few hours (acute soreness), or the soreness can be delayed for hours or even days after a training session (the technical term is "delayed onset of muscle soreness," or DOMS). DOMS is a result of structural damage to the muscle cells, and this damage happens mostly during eccentric or lengthening contractions. Not only do eccentric contractions produce soreness, but DOMS also slows the rate at which muscle glycogen is resynthesized.

Some DOMS early in a training program is necessary, as it maximizes the training response (remember that old coaching line: "you have to break muscles down before you rebuild them"?), and soreness will eventually be reduced during subsequent bouts of training. DOMS tends to be more prominent following resistance or power training than after endurance training. Resistance training requires significant eccentric contractions, while the eccentric component of running is much less prevalent. Plus, the muscle fiber types used in weight lifting have varying resistance to fatigue. Fast-twitch muscle fibers are recruited during resistance training (short-term explosive exercises), and these fibers fatigue much faster than their slow-twitch counterparts. Also during weight training, the exercise is localized to specific muscle groups, whereas aerobic training, like running, spreads the work (and subsequent soreness) over a much larger muscle mass.

The recovery process and subsequent adaptations permit the next bouts of training to be performed to a higher level. New muscle proteins are formed, increasing muscle strength. Glycogen stores in muscle are increased, as is the amount of enzymes involved in the anaerobic and aerobic production of energy. There are many other adaptations that occur within the body during recovery following exercise.

Over a period of time, training eventually produces a fitter, stronger, faster, and more powerful athlete. If too much time elapses between training sessions, however, then the training benefits are soon lost, and the athlete can even lose some of what has been achieved. If the recovery period is too short, there hasn't been sufficient time for adaptation. Low-intensity aerobic training can be structured into a training program in order to help boost recovery in between strenuous training sessions. This light exercise is sometimes called "active recovery" (in the soccer community it's called "regeneration training"), and it helps the recovery process through increasing the blood flow through muscles, which in turn enables the efficient removal of any lingering waste or breakdown products that may hinder the recovery process. If recovery is not an integral part of the training program, the body does not have a chance to build on the training already performed because physiological improvements only occur when the body is resting. If the principle of recovery is not followed, it is common for athletes to develop overuse injuries or even mild viral infections or experience the overreaching or overtraining syndromes.

Staleness, Overreaching, Overtraining, and Underperformance

The consequence of too little recovery time between training sessions, or too many high-intensity sessions performed in a short period of time, is "overtraining." I hear coaches talking about teenagers playing up to 140 games a year. How can you keep your interest playing nearly 3 games a week? Overtraining is a psychophysiological problem in which performance declines in spite of continued training. Fatigue is an unavoidable consequence of exercise and training. During periods of overtraining, however, levels of physical and psychological fatigue become much more pronounced, and underperformance is the consequence.

A reduction in performance in spite of increased training is the primary sign of overtraining. The physiological consequence is muscle damage, as muscles that do not recover between training bouts end up working in a compromised state. Muscle damage can be manifested as muscle soreness, earlier onset of fatigue, muscle pain, stiffness, or a higher than normal blood lactate level. Muscle damage from overtraining also impairs the ability of the muscles to restore glycogen, which reduces the amount of available fuel for the next bouts of exercise. Basically, the body begins to break down and fails to fully recover in time for the next training session. Other symptoms of overtraining are sleep disturbances, nausea, and higher than normal heart rates and blood pressure. Along with performance decrements, a good indicator of overtraining is the heart rate response to standard exercise. If a player is overtrained, the heart rate will be higher than when the athlete is fit. As soon as the coach or athlete realizes that it is difficult to maintain the heart rate in the target zone, the wise coach should be very careful to reduce or avoid the stress of training. Many coaches of highly competitive teams have their players run a standard, paced run (e.g., a 7:30 mile or eight to ten runs of the yo-yo test), measure the heart rate when they finish, and record the results. This test is then repeated later in the season, and heart rates are checked again. Normally, the postexercise heart rates should be consistent or decline as the players get fitter. Another sign of overtraining is a consistent decrease or increase of the resting heart rate (as measured in the morning upon awakening) and could also be considered as a signal for infection.

If any of these symptoms occur, the coach needs to modify the training for that athlete. High-intensity training is strongly discouraged in the presence of any of these symptoms, as further high-intensity training will lead to further deterioration in performance. Symptoms of overtraining are highly individual and subjective, making them difficult to identify. The presence of any of the symptoms means the player is either training too hard or getting insufficient recovery time between workouts.

Athletes in an overtrained state are at an increased risk of infection, as training can also suppress normal immune function. A good way for the coach to find out if a player is becoming overtrained is to ask questions of the athlete: "Sleeping OK?," "Feel rested when you wake up?," "No? Must not be sleeping through the night, are you?" In a game like soccer, a player that needs rest may lie, fearing that days away from training might mean losing playing time. Giving the "right" answer will not give the coach the information needed to help the athlete. Of course, it is possible her body may make the decision for her when she gets sick due to her suppressed immune system.

The treatment of overtraining consists of either a significant reduction in training intensity or complete rest, but the best medicine for overtraining is prevention. Training should be structured to avoid overtraining. Adequate rest is an integral part of any training program. Remember:

- Mix low-intensity, regenerative sessions with medium- and high-intensity sessions.
- Try not to perform too many high-intensity sessions back to back.
- Get enough rest, taking adequate time to recover between workouts.
- Get a full night's sleep.
- Increase the training load slowly.
- Keep a training diary of the type of workout, duration, and perceptions of workout intensity (on a 1–10 scale).
- Keep a record of what you ate and how you felt while exercising.
- Eat a balanced diet low in fat and high in complex carbohydrates.
- Perform a variety of exercises.

Overtraining is a syndrome that coaches of individual sport athletes (like swimmers, distance runners, cross-country skiers, and cyclists) must be constantly concerned about. Thankfully, this syndrome in pretty rare (but not unheard of) in soccer and other team sports. It can, and does, occur in selected players on professional teams or other highly competitive teams.

More on Periodization

Simply stated, periodization is the overall training plan for a team. The concepts are applied to a calendar year but can be used to plan a season, a week, or single day. Periodization is a manipulation of training volume, training intensity, and technique training during the training period. Figure 2.5 shows the basic relationship between the three factors. The training year is divided into four phases. The new competitive season starts at the end of the previous year during a most important period called "active rest." During this period, players stay active, but they do activities other than soccer like cycling, swimming, hiking, tennis, or rollerblading. By staying active, the player retains some of her fitness, but the "active rest" period takes her away from the game where overexposure might lead to staleness. The active rest phase is also important mentally because it ensures that the player doesn't get bored by the game.

The next phase is the "preparatory" phase, where fitness is slowly built up. The emphasis here is on high-volume, low-intensity training (e.g., jogging). During this period the running distance shortens, while the pace increases. "Transition" is the period between the more aerobic preparatory phase and the initial training camp. Here, volume is reduced, and intensity is raised. For example, fartlek running would be a good choice for the early transition period.

As the transition period progresses, move into some long interval runs followed by shorter, harder intervals. The final few weeks before formal training camp might include a lot of repeat runs at a fast (but not sprint) pace, such as 100 yards in 15 seconds with a 45-second rest: the typical 1 to 3 work to rest formula for interval training. The 100-yard distance is for male adult players; decrease the running distance as needed for younger players and females. The idea is to run for 15 seconds at a fast, hard stride. Start out doing ten to twenty repetitions per day of these runs, and add five to ten each week. The total would be based on the ages and playing expectations of the players and team. An under-16 team might do twenty to twenty-five of these

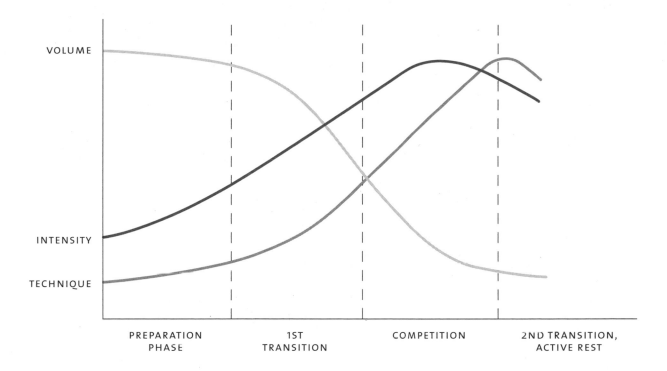

PREPARATION PHASE	1ST TRANSITION	COMPETITION	2ND TRANSITION, ACTIVE REST

repeat runs, while an adult, highly competitive player might work up to forty.

The "competition" phase is where the coach brings the players to match fitness with activities that closely mimic the game, and emphasis is placed on technique, tactics, and fitness. The total volume of running will be less than the preparation period, but the intensity will approach that necessary for the game.

Importance of Active Rest

The phase that is probably the most poorly understood is "active rest." Some players playing on multiple teams may never get an active rest period. For example, in some states soccer is a spring sport, and during the fall the school coach might have the team in the preparatory phase, while the club coach is in the competition phase. It's no wonder kids get burned out, injured, or sick.

Active rest is a critical phase for the physical development of the player. During this phase, the player should continue to be active but through other recreational sports and leisure activities. These more casual activities help players maintain a reasonable fitness level,

FIGURE 2.5
Conceptual Model for Periodization of Training

In the off-season, players need to maintain their fitness in preparation for the next season. The player has a responsibility to teammates to arrive in condition because being in shape prior to training camp means an easier transition to match intensity training and fewer injuries.

Many players decide only to play pick-up games to prepare for the season. Two reasons make pick-up games a poor choice for fitness training. First, these games are not intense enough; competitive games will be far more intense. Second, the off-season is the time to be doing other forms of training to prepare for more intense soccer-specific training.

Specifically, the off-season is the time to put in some mileage, and one of my favorite ways is to run on unpaved trails. Why trails? There are several reasons:

- Running trails is interesting. The scenery changes with nearly every step—you can't say that about running the streets, where it's house after house after house. Get out in the woods at the right time, and you are likely to see deer, fox, or more, depending on where you live.
- The solitude is invigorating. Leave the music at home and just listen to nature. Music might help you maintain pace on the streets, but pace is not your concern on the trails. Besides, you want to be able to hear that deer running away or that biker coming up behind you.
- Running trails is running as learning. Running the streets is endurance training, and that is fine. Running the trails is very different. Every step is an adventure and requires adjustment as you change stride length and frequency and foot placement to avoid obstacles like rocks and roots and prepare for landings on unsure footing. You have to decide where and how to plant virtually every footstep for a stable landing. Soon, you will plot out your steps three, four, or more steps ahead to avoid obstacles. What you are learning is how to control your push-off and landing while running and how to place your feet on the ground as you rotate your foot to avoid poor footing; you also learn how long your legs are, how big your feet are, and how much you have to bend over to avoid a branch. After a while, you will be planning your movements farther and farther ahead, sort of like planning your passing and running options one, two, or more passes ahead. Everything has some relation to the game. Need another reason? Trail running is probably the most widely used form of distance running by the Brazilian team.
- Hills are usually short and steep. Charge that hill for short, high-intensity running and the strength that it requires. Downhill can be very steep, and you have to control your body on every aspect of every step. This increases your control of your body, absolutely critical to landing from a jump or planting your foot to change direction. (Poor control in these areas is how players get noncontact injuries like knee and ankle injuries.) On really steep downhill stretches, don't be so proud that you can't walk down for a safer transition.
- But watch out, *trail running is dangerous*. Roots and rocks can trip you up, or if you land poorly you can sprain an ankle or be knocked off balance into a

tree. Running shoe companies make trail running–specific shoes that offer better support than routine jogging shoes. Best to run with a friend. And maybe that root really is a snake!

Go ahead and play those pick-up games for fun and to try out new techniques and tactics; they're just not for fitness.

while giving them time for psychological and emotional rest away from soccer.

Adaptation to training follows a predictable model. At the onset of training, there is a slight drop-off in performance due to things like muscle soreness and stiffness (the alarm phase). With time and exposure to training, the body begins to adapt to the new demands (the resistance phase). Training is manipulated to maintain fitness (the competition phase). If training continues to be increased even as performance declines, the athlete may slip into detraining (the exhaustion or overtrained phase). Once performance plateaus, back off training volume and intensity before beginning to ramp the training up again (the transition and preparation phases). Done properly, a new, higher level of performance is the result (the new, higher competition phase). I wish I had a formula to achieve this process, but there isn't one. Every player responds a bit differently to training.

OFF-SEASON TRAINING

Soccer, like most sports, is seasonal: there are periods of preparation (preseason, or preparation/transition), competition (in-season), and recovery (off-season or active rest). Preseason and in-season training belong to the coach. In the off-season it is the player's responsibility to complete the fitness program the coach has provided. What players do in the off-season will impact their performance in the next season. As I've stated several times in this book, it is easier to stay in shape than it is to get in shape. Most players, however, don't know how to maintain their fitness without a coach to supervise them, and most certainly have no clue what to do unless the coach lays it all out for them.

Maybe I'm getting old (true) and have some leftover ADHD (likely), but running long, slow distances is hard for me to do. I like distraction—no matter what I'm doing. While I'm typing this, I'm listening to music . . . loud music.

So when I go to run the streets, I prefer to run fartlek. The term is Swedish for "speed play," and the technique is quite easy to do but is more intense than normal jogging. For fartlek training, plan out a routine jogging course and leave your watch at home. Once you have adjusted to the run and have reached a steady state (maybe 3–5 minutes for you, 8–10 minutes for me), pick out a landmark ahead like the third driveway, the fourth telephone pole—anything. Then increase your running pace to that landmark. Don't sprint; just run faster than you were jogging. When you reach the landmark, slow down back to the pace you think you were running (the key word there is "think"), and continue at that pace until your breathing has recovered. Then pick out another landmark and repeat. After mul-

tiple days of fartlek training three things happen. First, the faster runs will get longer and longer (or faster for the same distance). Second, the time between the faster runs will become shorter and shorter because you will recover more quickly. Finally, your jogging pace between the harder runs will get faster and faster. All of these are signs of improved fitness. Fartlek running deals with perception of running pace. Remember, don't use a watch to manage your pace.

Fartlek running is best done in the off-season, though you could do this one or two days if your game schedule has maybe a 10-day break between matches. In the off-season, players should do a few weeks of basic long slow distance. The next week or two, they might replace two jogging days with two fartlek days. The next week or two, do three fartlek sessions (on nonconsecutive days). The player is now ready to increase his intensity, moving up to interval or repeat runs in the final preparation for training camp.

Proper Planning of Year-Round Training

Planning out the details of a training program requires an understanding of the periodization concept. Endurance can be trained by endurance training that is not specific to soccer, like jogging, cycling, and swimming. These types of activities would be performed during active rest and the start of the preparation phase. Endurance training is often neglected as a method to develop fitness in soccer. "We aren't training endurance runners" is what a coach might say. But we are training people to recover on the field during a match—recovery is an aerobic activity—and, in the absence of a team, aerobic fitness is developed on the streets and trails. In between competitive seasons, players should be encouraged to participate in endurance exercises like cycling, in-line skating, cross-country skiing, swimming, or hiking, in order to at least maintain and preferably improve fitness. Yes, the genetic component of endurance ability is a chief factor. However, this training should not be neglected. Endurance exercise not only develops fitness level, but it also mentally distracts the player from the "addiction" to playing. For speed and agility, practice other ball sports just for the joy of playing (such as badminton, tennis, squash, and playing five-a-side football; one of my favorites in the off-season was taking a soccer ball into a handball court), which may result in an improved fitness level while maintaining agility. These training activities should be recreational, never competitive.

Other Off-Season Considerations

Calorie intake. Since training volume is reduced during the off-season (fewer days per week and/or minutes per day), fewer calories will be burned. To maintain their weight during a period of reduced training, players will likely need to reduce their food intake. Some players may even need to lose weight to improve their performance. Don't make this decision without some good professional advice on whether weight loss is needed, and get advice on nutrition and weight-loss goals from a sports nutritionist. Most quality sports medicine clinics can direct you to one. Once the decision is made, the season for weight loss is the off-season, not the competitive season. Losing weight in-season puts the player on the express lane to poor performance and possible injury.

Strength training. Strength is one of the many factors of physical fitness, and in most cases, the stronger athlete is the better athlete. Strength training has some benefits that support the player in the game. For example, the stronger player will be able to resist physical challenges and be more resistant to injury. However, strength training doesn't really add all that much to kicking distance or shooting power. The best time to improve strength and power is the off-season. The coach should suggest activities that improve overall strength and not focus exclusively on the legs. Once the season begins, the goal of the weight room shifts from strength improvement to strength maintenance.

Rest. The soccer community has a real problem. Youth and professional players compete in too many games and have too few training sessions. When you add up school games, club team schedules, and in and out of season tournaments, some teenagers play 100 to 120 or more games a year. Training professionals suggest a ratio of training to games of 3–5 to 1 or higher, and the only real way to achieve such a ratio is to reduce the number of games. UEFA (Union of European Football Associations) did a study on injuries and performance in national team players from their member nations that showed greater rates of injury and poorer performance in players who played the most matches and trained the least in preparation for the 2002 World Cup. For some, the only rest a player gets is when he is injured. For the professional player it has been suggested that domestic league games be limited to sixty or fewer per year to avoid the fatigue that leads to poor performance and injury. The problem is that the professional owner makes money only when the team competes. (This conflict is part of the eternal "club vs. country" debate—a debate that is starting to rear its head in U.S. basketball, but that is another matter.) Planned rest periods followed by a planned reestablishment of fitness for the next season are needed, even in countries where professionals may only have only 8 weeks between seasons.

Rest is important. Take time away, and be active, but be away from the ball. Rest recharges batteries in preparation for the push to the next season. Remember, time away does not mean time down. The fastest way to lose fitness is to reduce the intensity of training. No player wants to be out of shape for early games or be rusty on the ball. In the NCAA, early season tourneys can make or break a season before it even gets started. Players want to get on the field and start playing. There is nothing more aggravating than having to spend time off the field due to an injury. Many injuries can be prevented by some training prior to entering the field. Need proof?

THREE WAYS TO REDUCE INJURIES . . . PRACTICALLY GUARANTEED

Preseason Conditioning

I haven't gone into detail about research studies because the nitty-gritty of research sometimes can be tedious. But a recent study out of Cincinnati tracked the injuries of 300 girls, aged 15–18, over two high school seasons. About half of the girls participated in a 7-week preseason conditioning program, and the rest didn't. The training program consisted of endurance, strength, agility, and plyometric activities. An athletic trainer then recorded all injuries according to location (ankle, knee, thigh, and so on), type (sprain, strain, fracture, and more), and severity (out for how long) during the competitive season. The results were startling. There were a total of ninety-eight injuries, for an overall injury rate of 0.3 injuries per player per season. Let's say a team carries twenty-four players; these results suggest that each team in the project sustained about eight injuries, give or take.

Here is the really important finding. Of the ninety-eight injuries, only seven occurred in the group that participated in the conditioning program. In the trained group, there was one ACL (anterior cruciate ligament) tear (versus eight in the untrained group), two ankle sprains (versus twenty-one), and one pulled quad muscle (versus seven). Only one trained athlete had a season-ending injury (the ACL tear), yet there were eleven season-ending injuries in the untrained group. About half of the injuries in the untrained players happened during practice, yet five of the seven injuries to the trained players occurred during games. How much more proof should coaches need? *The easiest and best way to prevent injuries is simply to improve the fitness of the players prior to the season.* Medical professionals in multiple sports will say that fitness is probably the best way to prevent injuries. Of course, in some sports (specifically American football), improved fitness has reduced some injuries while increasing others; the profile of injuries has changed.

Skill Level

Most studies detail the location, type, severity, and rate of injuries. A group of Norwegians added a skill factor to their project. Each coach was asked to grade the overall skill of each player, and the researchers then tracked injuries and reported the injuries based on players' skill level. While most experienced coaches might already have figured this out intuitively, the most skilled players were the least injured, and those with the poorest skill were the most frequently and most severely injured. There is a reasonable trade-off for skill training in the weeks prior to training.

It is important for the upcoming season to improve endurance and body control by doing lots of activities that will improve both. The healthier the players and the team, the more likely the team will have its best players on the field and hopefully a more successful season.

Don't Come Back Too Soon after an Injury

It should be obvious: do not return to competition until fully healed from an injury. Yet players do it all the time. Pulled muscle? A day or two off, then back to play. Sprained ankle? A nuisance injury, out maybe a week. Took a knee in the thigh? Couple days, tops. Players will usually try to minimize an injury in order to get back on the field. But the literature on injury contains a very interesting and extremely important finding: a major injury is very often preceded by an incompletely healed minor injury. That previous injury puts a player at risk for having that injury again. Strain a hamstring? The risk of another strained hamstring goes up by a factor of seven. A groin strain? The risk goes up by nearly six times. An ankle sprain? A knee sprain? Each goes up by about a factor of five. That nuisance ankle sprain should be protected for 6–12 months after an injury. You read that right: *6–12 months*. Get a good ankle brace from a physical therapist or an orthopedist and use it. Ankle supports do not affect touch on the ball or agility. Those are just excuses not to wear them. Many basketball players use ankle braces, and the agility demands of basketball exceed those of soccer. Ankle sprains are not to be minimized or ignored. As the ankle is the most commonly injured joint in soccer, an early return is placing the rest of the body at risk for something worse.

APPLYING TRAINING CONCEPTS TO SOCCER PRACTICE

The Dilemma of Physical Training and Match Schedule

As a season beckons, coaches are eager to plan out the season. Books and videos of skills, drills, and games are studied, selected, discarded, and reconsidered until finally every minute of each training session is filled. More planning, however, is yet to be completed. Remember, the prime variables of training are the frequency of training (days per week), the intensity of training, and the duration of training (minutes per day). In many cases, the frequency is somewhat fixed. A school program might train/play daily (five days a week, as three training days and two games or four training days and one game), while a youth club team might train twice a week and play one or two games over the weekend. You don't have unlimited training time, and yet you somehow have to cram in technical skill training, team tactics, and fitness. The smart coach will figure out how all this should be managed before the season begins.

Probably, the first thing to do is set up a 4-week calendar with six game dates. First, cross off game dates. Next, everyone knows it is better not to train hard on the day before a game, so cross off the six days before a game. Many teams and leagues restrict training on Sundays, so cross off the four Sundays. So far, we've crossed off 16 days. Now, most coaches know that it is important to hold what many call "regenerative training" on the day after a game, so cross off these six days (22 total days are now crossed off). Finally, I hope that from reading this book you will realize that it is not advisable to train hard (hard, soccer-specific training) on two consecutive days. Where there are two consecutive open days, cross off one of the two days. How many days are left for fitness work? You might have only three or so days in the whole month that could be devoted to fitness. You might wonder how fitness is improved during the season. It should be no surprise that when the endurance of soccer players is followed over a season, there is little change after the first third of the season. The bulk of improvement in fitness happens in the first third of the season (beginning with the first day of training camp), then fitness levels are maintained for the rest of the season. Some studies have even shown a decrease in fitness toward the end of the season.

One last thing to remember about schedules like this: For those who play, the competitive game "counts" as fitness training. In the NCAA, games are fairly rigidly scheduled, with games on Thursdays and Saturdays or Fridays and Sundays. This gives two hard sessions a week just from games. The smart coach then works her players pretty hard on Tuesdays, for a third day of hard training.

Organizing a Training Session for Fitness

By this point, I hope you are asking the question about organizing a specific session to stress fitness. I will offer some general guidelines because I know you don't want a cookbook.

Begin the session with a reasonable warm-up, usually consisting of fun, light activities to get the players moving. Once the players break a sweat, some flexibility exercises can be introduced. Also add

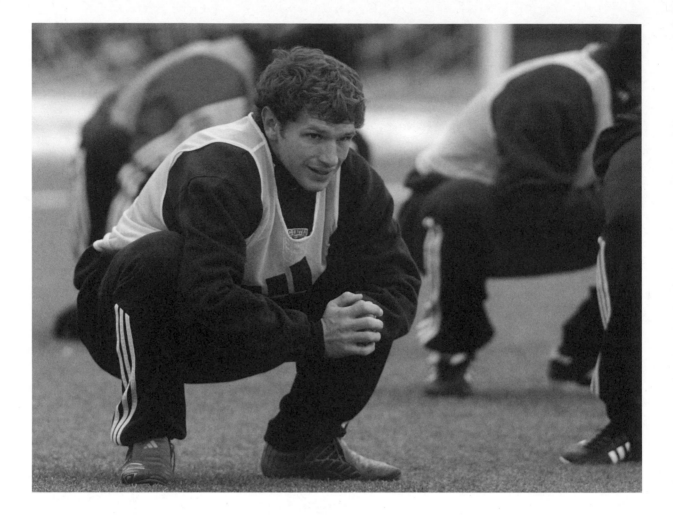

Justin Moose of the D.C. United, 2006. Any soccer player can develop soft tissue injuries in the groin. Special attention needs to be paid to this vulnerable area. Players can stretch by using their elbows to push their knees apart or strengthen the groin muscles by using their knees to push against their elbows as they apply resistance. (Photograph by Tony Quinn; SoccerStock.com)

some of those activities (like the F-MARC 11—see chapter 3) that aid in injury prevention. These will help prepare the players for further training activity and also teach valuable lessons on controlling their bodies.

Next, some individual ball skill training (very low intensity work) can be followed by small group work (e.g., 3v3, 4v4, 5v2, 6v4) at a higher intensity. These small group activities are taught ad infinitum at coaching clinics, and you probably have your favorites—keep away, two-touch keep away, grid drills, and games, things like that.

Large group work (as big as your team allows, up to perhaps 7v7 or 8v8) follows. Restrictions should be placed on the games so that the players have to run and think. This helps with their "game intelligence" and minimizes players' standing around. When I attended the U.S. Soccer Federation school way back when (when it was new), the instructors stressed that play should *never* go on without some restriction, to force the players to think, regardless of age. Restrictions can be technical (e.g., a player must trap and pass with the weak foot or always pass with the outside of the foot), tactical (e.g., on offense, attackers play with their backs to the goal—this teaches midfielders to come forward to shoot on goal; or "up-back-through," where a forward pass is dropped back and followed by a through pass to a teammate cutting between defenders), or fitness-related (e.g., two-touch speeds up the game; run 10 meters in any direction after any pass). Coaching books and schools teach endless variations.

Now, let's work out a session to focus on fitness, for one of those few "blank" days in the calendar I drew up. Choose almost any drill or small group game and modify it to stress any combination of fitness, technique, or tactics.

- *Low-intensity work*: Play 6v6 with goalkeepers on half a field with no restrictions for about 15 minutes (technical and tactical coaching is offered throughout).
- *Higher-intensity work*: Mark off a 20-meter zone across the middle of the field. The teams play six attackers versus five defenders in one end of the field with the sixth defensive player at the opposite end of the field. When the defensive team gets the ball, they pass directly to their far teammate, and all but one from the other team sprint across the midfield and play at the other end. The game continues back and forth across the no-play zone (some call this the "no midfield" game or "deep" game). Play this harder game for about 10 minutes.
- *Very high intensity work*: Still playing the 6v6 game, when the defenders get the ball and pass it across the midfield, they get two points for a goal (or one point for a shot on goal) if their entire team is in the new attacking area *and* at least one opponent (other than the one who is supposed to stay) is left behind. Play this very high intensity game for maybe 5 minutes.

Coaches don't need dozens of fitness activities. Choose a few that work, and repeat them on fitness days. Once a season starts, fitness days are limited, so it is unlikely that players will get bored doing the same few drills. Skill work, however, needs lots of variety.

Like all coaches, I read books on games to give my practices variety. Here are a couple of games that have become favorites of mine.

1. "Route 1 soccer" means direct play on a field that for all practical purposes is the width of a penalty area. You all have seen it. In a translation of a German book I came across was a game called a "winger's game." A cone was placed about 10 yards in from the sideline, level with the corner of the penalty area. The restriction was simple. The ball had to be passed or dribbled between the cone and the sideline (in the offensive end) before a shot could be taken. After a while, the team gets pretty good at looking to the side, rather than straight ahead, for that first outlet pass. I would use this game every practice to pound the concept into the heads of the players (this particular team was under-15). You can combine this game with other restrictions: all passes with the weak foot; or all passes with the outside of the foot; or first ball contact with the weak foot; or overlap every forward pass; or all crosses by the front runners (they have to make the diagonal run to get the ball and cross to midfielders coming up). You are only limited by your imagination. I would play these restricted games regardless of the size of the training game, from 4v4 all the way up to 11v11. Route 1 soccer is a good route to take; just don't take it every time down the field.

2. The set-up for this next game is simple—the execution is a killer—and you will see an unexpected outcome. Place a cone 10–15 yards in from each sideline on the midfield line (or wherever the midfield line would be when playing small-sided games on a smaller field). The restriction sounds simple enough: the ball crosses the midfield line between the cone and the sideline, and the players cross the midfield line between the cones. Think about that. No dribbling up the sideline. No dribbling up the middle of the field. No passes across the middle of the field. No clears. When you have the ball in your own end, you have to get the ball to the side, and then pass the ball up the line to a teammate making a diagonal run across the midfield line. When you first try this, the game will be stopped over and over and over because of rule violations. The players will get frustrated—very frustrated—at not being able to get going for all the stoppages. When they are finally successful, they will attack with abandon, but that is not the unexpected outcome. One of the hardest things for a young forward to learn is to go on immediate defense when the ball is lost. In this game, when the ball is lost, the team will work very, very hard (and be very vocal about it) to regain possession in the offensive end of the field so that they don't have to do that ridiculous restriction you set. Guaranteed.

3. This last game teaches counterattacks by playing the ball into space and encourages the goalkeeper to be ready to come out and intercept through balls, but this isn't kick-and-run. Simply play offsides like in ice hockey. In ice hockey the first thing across the blue line is the puck. Play any size game in terms of players or field size, but lay out a midfield line. When your team gets the ball, everybody has to be in the defensive end of the field. To attack, the ball is either dribbled across the midfield line or is passed into space for a player to run onto (no dumping into the corners as is so popular in ice hockey!). If you get tired of all the balls going out of bounds or being picked up by the goalkeeper or cen-

tral defender before a striker can run onto it, encourage the players to pass the ball toward the corner flag. Pass the ball too square, and the ball runs out of bounds on the side. Pass it too straight up the field, and the goalkeeper or central defender gets to it first. Teach the younger players to look for the flag or ask for the receiver to tell their teammate to aim for the flag. This game also teaches players how to apply the best pace on the pass for their teammate to catch up to the ball. The best restriction to add to this one is the number of passes to a shot. When on offense, for example, players only get three to four passes to a shot, or all passes to the shot must be a cross. Use your imagination.

Notice how the concept of periodization is applied to this session. The volume (time played) drops for each game, while the intensity is raised. Depending on the age and goals of the team, this series of games could be followed by small-sided activities, then some skills, and finally a cool-down. For more competitive teams, after a break the routine could be repeated as before, followed by some easier small-sided games, some light skill work, then a cool-down.

The "no midfield" game can be further modified. To speed up the transition to the other end of the field, make the midfield shorter (10 meters) for short, fast sprints. To encourage longer runs (and accurate long passes), increase the size of the midfield to 30 or 40 yards.

Of course, other technical or tactical restrictions can be added to make the game even harder. A game need not have just one restriction. Practice games of 11v11 with no restrictions are not good for fitness training. A typical possession in soccer involves four players and three passes or fewer; small-sided games (4v4) are very good for teaching general tactics with many ball contacts.

Special Considerations When Planning Training

Relationship between intensity and duration. Players can't train hard *and* long. If you get nothing else out of this book, remember this: Intensity is inversely related to duration; the harder one works, the less time one can maintain that intensity. Trying to work long and hard without rest (or low-intensity days) leads to a substantial risk of overuse injuries and possibly underperformance or overtraining.

Rate of improvement in fitness. Figure 2.6 displays this relationship graphically. Yes, a player can work his way into condition in a short

FIGURE 2.6

Relationship between Rate of Improvement in Fitness and Eventual Level of Fitness

Note: Line A shows that a player can work his way into condition in a short amount of time, but his ultimate level of fitness will be low and the time he can maintain that level of fitness will be brief. Line B indicates that achieving fitness more slowly leads to higher levels of fitness that can be maintained longer.

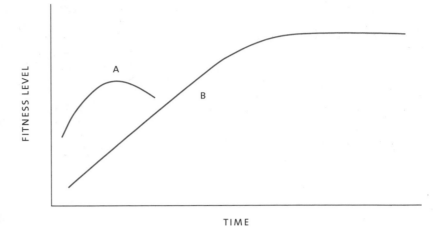

time, but the ultimate level of fitness will be low, and the length of time he can maintain that fitness will be brief (line A). If fitness is developed more slowly, higher levels of fitness will be achieved, and those levels can be maintained longer (line B).

Improvement in running (not sprinting) speeds. If you train by walking, you become better at walking. If you jog, you get better at jogging *and* walking. If you train at progressively faster speeds (but not sprinting speeds), you improve your ability to run at the fastest speed and all speeds below. That is why repeated, longer (like 75–100 meters) runs at a hard, but not maximal, pace are good. Male professional players sprint only about 800–1,000 meters (of 10,000 meters total) in a game (less for younger ages and competitive levels), so they cover about 90% at speeds below a sprint. In the final weeks prior to training camp, run a lot at this hard stride (those repeated 15-second runs talked about earlier), and you will get better at those fast speeds and all the speeds below.

Economical training. Coaching schools teach the concept of "economical training." You've read that all sports are a combination of fitness, technique, and tactics. Economical training means combining two or all three into one activity. My coaching improved dramatically once I learned this concept.

How often must high-intensity training be performed? Most training specialists feel that three nonconsecutive high-intensity training sessions a week need to be scheduled. Remember that a competitive game is considered intense training. Playing one game a week means

One of the most important topics developed at coaching schools is the concept of economical training. Soccer is a combination of fitness (physical and psychological), technique, and tactics. The instructors take great pains to show how two or more of these concepts can be trained within one drill, and drills that fit the bill are shown in dozens of coaching books. The soccer concept of economical training is probably one of the most important models that new coaches can take home to their players. I know my coaching skills improved dramatically after I attended the U.S. Soccer coaching school, having learned about "economical training."

However, the concept of economical training has a limitation: only so much intensity can be built into a ball game. Yes, intensity is highest when one is in control of the ball, and yes, small-sided games offer the most opportunity for ball contact and thus intensity. The key aspect is the ball. When one player has the ball, the rest of the players do not. Restrictions can keep them busy, but still, due to the nature of the game, ball contact is brief and infrequent. No one is working as hard as the player with the ball, and that player may only work hard for a few seconds and have a long time to recover before the next possession.

So, if you want real economical training designed to increase fitness, where you can train an entire team at once, interval training is the ticket. I have routinely said that soccer players don't know what serious, intense training involves, as a rower or a 400-meter hurdler might. I also joke that when it comes to training, if the distance is longer than the length of the field and doesn't involve the ball, soccer players want nothing to do with it. But coaches and trainers of the truly elite teams know that there is only so much one can achieve with the ball. To develop a huge fitness reserve to call on in a game, sometimes traditional track-style interval training must be considered. I have a British colleague who was once a competitive 800-meter runner. He had the opportunity to do some work with Real Madrid and said it was the first soccer team he had ever seen that worked what he considered "hard." At one session, the players did repeat 400-meter runs at a strong pace, then did typical soccer training followed by a series of 200-meter repeats, all at a pace far in excess of what soccer requires. If you get the chance to see an elite team in residence during their preparatory period, you might just see track-style workouts.

two intense sessions should be scheduled. If there are two games, then one hard day would be scheduled. Many club teams train twice a week and play one or two games over the weekend. The game is considered a training stimulus, so in order to get three days of hard training, there must be some high-intensity work scheduled for each training session.

Players should arrive in some measure of fitness. These comments focus on mostly the high school and older player. When a player arrives for the first day of team training, she should have some level of fitness. The problem is most players don't have the experience to develop a training program for the weeks prior to training camp. They could be directed to the English FA (Football Association) website for a couple of good programs. Or they could follow a specified program that a coach has developed. The U.S. Youth Soccer Association (USYSA) or National Soccer Coaches Association of America (NSCAA) annual meetings usually have presentations on training programs. A favorite of mine is the "repeat 100s," which I've mentioned earlier. Players run (not sprint) 100 yards (up the sideline of a football field) in about 15 seconds and then take 45 seconds to walk to the other sideline. They start the next run when the recovery time is up, ready or not. A player could start out with a week of two sets of ten, then add five runs each week. I have seen players (male collegiate) run up to fifty per session. This exercise trains recovery from hard running. The total distance at this speed is greater than what is covered in games, but it does help develop a substantial reserve for competition. In another program a player trots 100 yards, turns around and jogs 100 yards, turns around and runs hard for 100 yards, turns around and walks that 100 yards, then repeats. If players arrive with some measure of fitness, the coach's job, then, is to bring the team and players to match fitness. Simply playing matches is not sufficient preparation for training camp.

How much of a training session should be devoted to high-intensity training? People who study training suggest that no more than one-third of the sports-specific training (i.e., not the warm-up, cool-down, etc.) should be devoted to high-intensity work. Let's assume that once warm-up and supplemental activities have been done, the plan is for 90 minutes of training. The coach should have the training divided into low-, moderate-, and high-intensity portions. Don't put all the high-intensity work into one 30-minute segment because the players will be tired during the final 10–15 minutes and won't work as hard as they should. So, divide the training time in half (two 45-minute periods). Now devote about 15–20 minutes to low-intensity work (ball skills, small-group activities, some unrestricted scrimmage). Next, increase the intensity for about 15 minutes, followed by 15 minutes of the highest-intensity work planned for that day. Now take a break, and

The English FA (Football Association) is among the few governing bodies that are really proactive in coaching education. Outside of the United States (in the United States, the National Soccer Coaches Association of America, or NSCAA, is the largest soccer coaches' association in the world—if you are a coach and not a member, you should be) and Canada, most of the coaching education and preparation takes place in Western Europe. Many other countries don't stress coaching education; they rely on talent. The FA has a sport sciences program that is about the most comprehensive program going. The courses it offers extend beyond just skills and tactics. For example, the FA runs a continuing audit of injuries among professional players in an attempt to make the game safer. Its journal publications are fascinating (for those of you who are interested, search the PubMed database with the search terms "Hawkins RD" and "soccer" for the relevant articles). The FA also offers a variety of courses devoted to soccer fitness. Check out the website at <www.TheFA.com>. It's a fun way to kill some time.

I don't like to outline a canned program simply because all teams, programs, situations, and players have unique circumstances. I prefer to pass along the concepts and let the coaches prepare their training for their teams. The FA, however, has prepared two very good programs—one 3 weeks long, the other 6 weeks long—that you might want to look at. To see the programs, go to <www.theFA.com>, click on the "Grassroots" tab, and select "Preseason Training."

then start the ramp all over again. The players will get far more out of the hard work as two 15-minute segments than as one 30-minute segment.

Specificity of training. This concept was discussed more fully earlier in this chapter. Many coaches mistakenly assume that the way to learn how to play 11v11 is to play 11v11. In earlier comments on the nature of the game I pointed out that the real essence of the game, meaning when a team is in possession of the ball, is not 11v11 but 4v4. Well over 90% of all possessions begin and end in three passes (and four players) or less. Thus, there is some real rationale behind all the 4v4 games in coaching books. The Dutch are some of the biggest proponents of 4v4 training. I recall that in my last year of coaching college we never (you read that right, *never*) played 11v11 in training. All tactical training was done as 4v4 up to 8v8. When a match finally came around, each player had experienced all aspects of what was essentially positionless soccer, and they were so hungry for 11v11 that

At a women's national team camp prior to the 1996 Atlanta Olympics, I watched a number of training sessions, most of which no one in his right mind would do voluntarily: they were tough! One game in particular caught my eye. The players were divided into four-player teams, plus a goalkeeper (even Coach Tony DiCicco had to play). They played for maybe 10–15 minutes and kept score. At a short break, winning teams were noted (each player on the winning team got a "W"), new opponents were set, and off they went again. After another 10–15 minutes, the results were recorded and so on, until they had played a round-robin with all the teams. Goalkeepers stayed on the same field, and their records were kept separately. The following week, they did the same thing but with different team rosters. The results for each player were kept and posted. The idea was that the best players (i.e., "winners")

would have the best records. I liked that: competition, 4v4, the barest essentials of the game.

It reminded me of a similar practice used in rowing called "seat races." Rowers get put into four-oared shells with a coxswain. They race some distance, maybe 1,000 meters. The winners are noted, with each rower in the shell getting a "W." One rower is swapped between two boats, and they race back, with results noted again. The idea is that the rowers who can really pull the shell will show up in the winning boats over and over.

Some ice hockey teams do something sort of similar but during games. It's called the plus/minus. If you are on the ice when your team scores, you get a plus, but if you are on the ice when the opponents score, you get a minus. As the season rolls on, if the minuses outnumber the pluses, you get moved "down" the roster and get less playing time.

they played with abandon. Of course, maybe that was just the situation and those players, but if I were to go back the sidelines, I would certainly try it again.

The easiest way to add intensity. The easiest way to increase intensity is to simply add the ball. At all running speeds, the requirement of running is increased by 10–15% when dribbling. Therefore, to increase intensity, add a ball; the more opportunities there are for a player to control the ball, the harder the work will be. Small-sided games are the best for this purpose because there is far more opportunity to be on the ball. You might think that the easiest game here is one my players used to call "burn 'em." You can guess the restriction—beat a player with a dribble before passing. What happens is the others end up standing around while one tries to find someone to beat. You have to be creative and add rules to limit standing on this one.

The best way to train at very high intensity. Two words: interval training. Get to know a track coach.

Weight Training

Improved strength is a very valuable commodity in modern soccer. The major portion of the work should be done outside of the competition phase, still following the principles of periodization. During the season, weight training is continued, but as a maintenance program, not an improvement program. Your new best friend should be someone like a strength coach at a college or a personal trainer who has worked with team sports.

Flexibility Training

A warm muscle is more receptive to flexibility training. Also, flexibility training, being important but low-intensity work, should be continued even during the active rest period of the year. Just be sure that a warm-up is done before the flexibility work. Coaches, please remember that *flexibility is not warm-up*, no matter when you did it when you were young. Once a sweat begins, the body is warm enough to begin flexibility training.

Considerations for Youth

There are many studies that demonstrate the trainability of children (i.e., those under 10 years old). Train a child for fitness and his or her fitness improves along the lines of adolescents, teenagers, and adults. In a ball game that requires skill development for success, many coaches focus on skills. Plus, many leagues allow unlimited substitution, so the emphasis on match fitness is less important as players generally don't play the entire match. My opinion: the very young (elementary school age) would be losing valuable skill time should emphasis be placed on fitness at the expense of skills.

Don't Ever Forget

Training programs will not eliminate the perception of training intensity. The individual perception of a given training load is important. If signals of fatigue or overtraining appear, the training program must be modified for the individual player. In particular, high-intensity

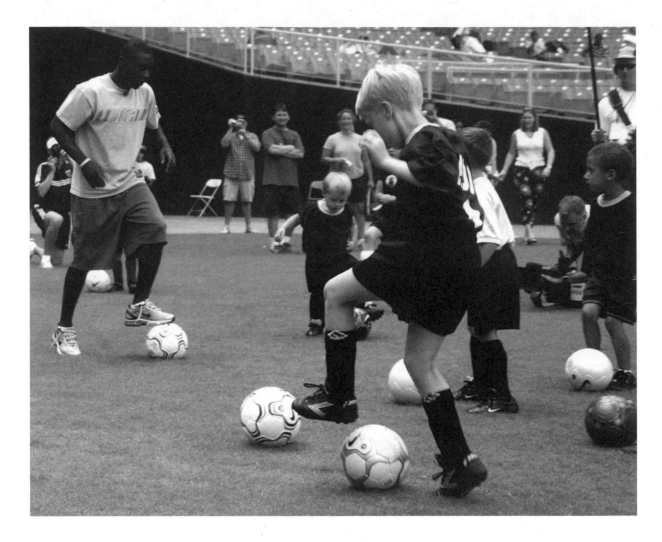

Freddy Adu trains young soccer players at the America Scores Clinic, 2004. Young players work on skills by imitating what they see, then trying it on their own. That's why at least one coach needs to be skilled. (Photograph by Tony Quinn; SoccerStock.com)

training should not to be performed when the coach identifies signs of excess fatigue or overtraining. Due to the high frequency of games, general fatigue and overtraining are continuous threats to the fitness level of any player. Still, underperformance is sometimes thought to be due to a lack of training. In some cases this perception may indeed be correct, yet in other players the opposite is true. Rest days or low-intensity regenerative training sessions often have a much better impact on fitness and performance levels than an increased training load. Therefore, if the player feels unable to continue the prescribed training program due to fatigue, the coach should be contacted. If this isn't done, the training program may actually be detrimental to performance.

TRAINING

- Always start each training session with a regular warm-up and end the session with a cool-down (including the stretching program).
- For those athletes who have a midweek game, it is very important (1) to do regenerative training the day after a match and (2) to do a light training session the day before a game, including a good warm-up, mobilization exercises, stretching, and speed exercises. Ideally, this training session should be done on the field on which the game is to be played.
- When performing high-intensity training sessions, the running time should be such that the player can run at a high intensity but still be able to maintain the speed for several exercise periods. The coach should ensure that the exercise intensity during high-intensity training sessions does not become so high that the training becomes exclusively speed-endurance training. If the intensity is too high, the player will not be able to keep a high enough work rate during subsequent work periods, and the desired effect of this high-intensity training will be lost. Access to a heart rate monitor (e.g., Polar HeartWatch) is very helpful for determining intensity.
- Give the players an off-season fitness program so that they will show up for preseason training camp with a degree of fitness that they can improve to a higher level and maintain for a longer time. Don't assume the players can figure out a program on their own. If players can improve during the off-season every year, their basic endurance will be a little better each year, which can make a substantial difference over a career.
- Train them as well as possible in the preseason, and try to maintain this preseason level through the season by following the suggestions made in this chapter. While fitness can be achieved in a short preseason period, the ultimate level of fitness will stay low and can only be maintained for a short period of time.
- You may be able to keep training the team harder as the season progresses. To do this, plan the season around the fitness plan while ignoring some parts of the game schedule, especially at the beginning of the season. When I was young, a coach called this training through a game. Yes, it can be risky if the team is tired and playing a very motivated team.

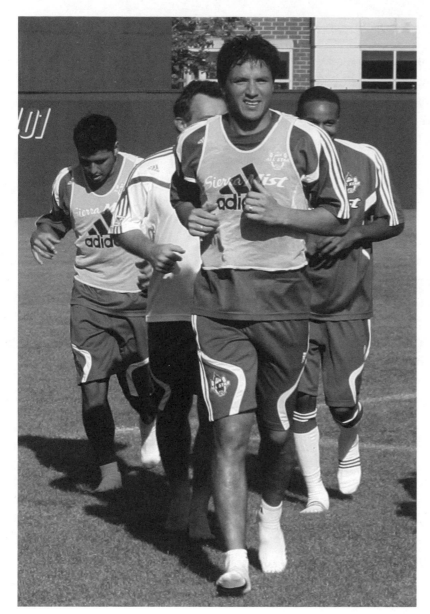

A slow, postplay jog is an important part of a cool-down. Note that these players have removed their studded footwear. Soccer shoes are made to play with a ball and should be worn only when a ball is involved. On a nice field like this one, players can jog wearing only socks. Have a pair of running shoes handy for all non-ball-related running. (Photograph by Tony Quinn; SoccerStock.com)

• Competitive games count as a training day, but only for those who actually play. In this regard, equal opportunity should be provided for sports participation. I remember watching São Paulo FC playing one night. The next day I was lucky enough to go to team training. On the field were the players who hadn't played or dressed the night before (the team carries about thirty players), and they were going through regular training. Those who had played the night before were doing a regenerative pool workout and never even stepped on the field.

- Training leads to two major adaptations in the body. The first is the ability of the cardiovascular system to deliver oxygen to the muscle cells, and the second is the ability of the muscle cells to use the delivered oxygen. Research shows that the central cardiovascular system's ability to deliver oxygen to the muscles improves slowly, while the muscle cells improve their ability to use the delivered oxygen pretty quickly; when training is stopped, the muscle cells lose most of what they have gained fairly fast (10 days to 2 weeks is about right), but the cardiovascular system detrains slowly. Most of us probably have experienced this when working out after being off for a short break. That first workout doesn't feel too bad. During that workout, the cardiovascular system takes up the slack from the cells that detrained so quickly. However, lay off for a month or more, and players start back from zero when it comes to endurance fitness.

With this rather long discussion about fitness, you might be asking something like, "Is my team fit?" About the only way to determine fitness is to analyze players through a variety of tests. There are many different ways to test, and some can be very expensive. But in the end, testing comes down to lab versus field-based tests.

Lab versus Field Testing

The essential difference between the two types of testing is that lab tests measure specific components of fitness, and field tests estimate what one might get from a lab test. Lab tests require expensive equipment and technical expertise to administer and interpret, plus it requires a long time to fully test a team, as you only test one player at a time. Field tests generally need simple things like a stopwatch and a measuring tape. Lab tests give results of endurance in units like milliliters of oxygen per kilogram of body mass per minute of work. In general, while the units are cumbersome, the higher the number the better the endurance. A lab test of endurance might be done on a treadmill at a set speed, with the incline being increased every cou-

There are a number of reasons that I favor fitness testing:

1 Determination of fitness status: I have said over and over in this book that the player must shoulder some of the responsibility for his or her fitness level by training before the season begins. Testing at the start of training camp is a sure way to see just who has done their training homework. You think the U.S. men's 2004 Olympic gold-medal heavyweight eights in rowing weren't tested when they arrived for training camp (and repeatedly throughout training)? Fitness goals for players and teams can also be set.

2 Training adaptation: Throughout a season or a year, fitness comes and goes depending on what players are doing. You can easily document just how much players have gained through training (and assess just how well you think your players are progressing, fitness-wise). Plus, you can also determine how much a player has lost due to injury by checking her fitness during rehabilitation. For example, recovery from a sprained medial collateral ligament (in the knee) can be as long as 12 weeks. Is your central midfielder ready to play a full 90 minutes in her first game? If her beep test is close to her previous tests, maybe.

3 Positive feedback: As players improve, they like to know just how much better they are doing. Some objective proof that they have improved their endurance or recovery rates is good motivation. The biggest changes will be seen in endurance and fatigue levels when doing repetitive speed tests; change will be less obvious for agility and vertical jump tests.

Two things fitness testing should not be used for:

1 Testing for testing's sake: Tests of fitness should be used to modify training. If the results are just going to fill some folder, don't waste everyone's time.

2 Testing should *never* be done and the results *never* used for punitive measures: Absolutely never test, find a player lacking in some factor, and then punish him with training or embarrass him in front of teammates because of poor results. There is a fine line between using test results for punishment and for motivation. Anson Dorrance posts fitness test scores (and lots of other scores) for motivation and to foster a competitive attitude. This is not the same as berating a player for poor fitness.

ple of minutes, until the player says, "I'm done." (This is a test we all should do at least once in our lives. Run 'til you drop—think about that.) During the test, all expired air is collected and analyzed for volume, oxygen, and carbon dioxide. In my mind, while the number is important, the most important factor is how long the test lasted (everybody does the same test). Most think their VO_2 max is a critical number, and it is. However, consider this scenario: Two players have a vo_2 max of 60 milliliters/kilograms/minute (typical for elite adult male soccer players), but the first player stops the test at 9 minutes, and the second player stops at 12 minutes. Who has the better endurance? The second player, who has the same vo_2 max but more time on the test. The first player was exhausted at 9 minutes but the second player was only two-thirds of the way through his test and had lots of reserve left in the tank. Play that guy in the midfield!

While lab tests are the gold standard for measuring various factors of fitness, field tests are far more practical, cheaper, more time-efficient, and easier to interpret. An entire team can be tested in a single practice.

Field Tests

What I'll describe is a series of tests done on soccer players, with the averages for youth and adult players who have taken these tests. As you might have guessed from comments throughout this book, I do not recommend testing elementary school–age players, as fitness is not a major concern for children that young because of substitution and guaranteed-play guidelines for most youth leagues.

Speed. As simple as the concept of speed is, testing it is a challenge. In running, the components are the reaction time to the starter, acceleration, top speed, and holding the speed for as long as possible. It all depends on what you want to know. Because some sprint test distances are very short and fitness improvements are measured in tenths of a second, many people either use a test that combines all features of speed (like a 30–50 yard sprint) or take a big leap and have the club invest in electronic timing. These devices can run as high as $1,000, but they are a very sound investment, darn near indestructible, and have numerous uses beyond this simple test. (For example, they are a whole lot more practical than a radar gun that lots of clubs think is important for measuring shot speed. In my opinion, the gun is for little more than bragging rights, but I digress.)

- *30–50 yard (or meter) sprint*: Simply measure out the distance, get a couple of stopwatches, have a parent signal the start (usually with arm motion), and time the full sprint. Each player should probably get at least two, but preferably three, trials. Keep either the best or

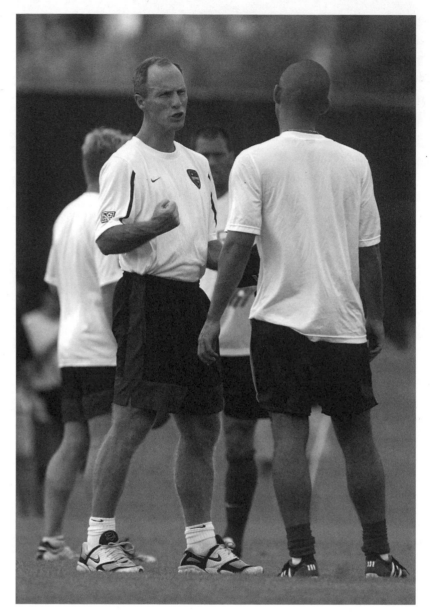

Major League Soccer coach Bob Bradley, 2003. At a coaching course, I once said to an instructor, "So, if I'm on the sideline at practice" and was immediately stopped and firmly told, "At practice, you are always on the field, never on the sidelines." (Photograph by Tony Quinn; SoccerStock.com)

the average of the two fastest trials. Test a group first, then repeat to give players a chance to recover between runs.

• *7 x 30 meter sprints*: As I state throughout this book, soccer-specific fitness is less about outright speed than about how quickly one recovers between runs. Soccer is played at high speeds and lower speeds, with recovery time between runs. So, with the aid of electronic timing (a must on this one), set up timers at the start, at 10

TRAINING

meters, and at 30 meters. The player sprints through the 30 meters as fast as possible, then trots back around to the start in 25 seconds (never a problem). Count down the last 5 seconds so the player knows when to start again. You will record two times from the electronic clocks: the 0–30 meter total sprint time with a 0–10 meter split. A 20-meter "flying" sprint (a 10-meter sprint with a 10-meter head start) is obtained by subtraction. These are obtained for all seven runs. After the times are collected, figure out the fastest sprint for all three distances (usually the first or second sprint); the average of all seven for each distance; and finally the fatigue for each distance (figured as percent decline: [slowest − fastest/ fastest] x 100). The slowest runs are usually the sixth or seventh run. Yes, this is a lot of data: three split times multiplied by seven sprints multiplied by however many players is a lot of sprint times. Spreadsheets are essential, as is care in inputting the numbers. And reducing all this data takes some time. If you don't know how to copy, paste, and sort on a spreadsheet, you will after having done this a time or two.

I tend to figure sprint speeds as meters/second as it makes more sense to me (10 meters/10-meter time for each distance). It takes a while to do a team in this test, as it takes around 3.5 minutes per player (30 seconds per sprint). When you get good at this, get two people to time the recovery and stagger two players (it doesn't take 30 seconds to write down the times). The first player sprints, the timers record the times, reset the timers, and signal ready, then the second player starts around 15 seconds into the first player's recovery period. A team can be done this way in half the time, though it takes practice and confidence in your timing methods. This test is a favorite of mine. The player with less than 10% fatigue in the three sprint speeds is plenty fit to compete. Test results for one boys' under-17 residential program *averaged* around 2% fatigue prior to an important competition, with numerous players showing no fatigue. Twenty-five seconds was plenty of time to recover fully between runs. The results can also give you some objective information on your team. For example, your fastest player on the 0–10 meter time is a player who gets up to speed quickly and is best suited for the shortest sprints, like a forward quickly sprinting past a defender, or a central defender covering that forward. The players with the fastest flying 20-meter sprint are probably best suited to put themselves in position to run onto balls played into space. So don't position them where they will receive mostly passes to feet. Rather, design their role to receive balls played into spaces. Those with the least fatigue will be able to give that speed over and over again.

Power. Power is the rate of force production. On the field this is usually measured as a vertical jump—and there are several different ways to measure vertical jump, differing mostly in how the player makes an approach to the jump. The simplest way is to have chalk dust in a bowl. The player dips a finger in the dust and touches a wall straight up over his head. Then he jumps and touches the wall at the top of the jump. The jump height is measured (in inches or centimeters) as the distance between the two marks. There is a cool device called a Vertec that lots of teams and schools have, which doesn't require the chalk or wall. There is also a mat called the Just Jump, which is a simple timing platform that times flight time (it's proportional to jump height). As I said, the approaches to the jump are varied, and your approach may be different from that of another team, but that is okay—just keep using the same method.

The first approach method is really no approach—it is a standing vertical jump. After the reach mark is placed on the wall, the player squats down and jumps as high as possible and touches the wall. The second method uses a one-step approach. The player takes one step back. When ready, she takes that step forward, leaps up (off two feet, not off one foot as in a layup), and touches the wall at the height of the jump. Always watch and make sure the player uses a two-foot takeoff. All vertical jump tests use a two-foot takeoff. The third method uses a three-step approach (and a two-foot takeoff). Obviously, the more steps, the higher the jump. Even more obvious, those with the highest vertical jumps are likely to be the best headers. Take the best of three jumps or the average of the two best of three trials.

Another test of power (or some might call it leg strength) is a standing triple jump. The player lines up on a starting line, feet comfortably apart, then does a standing long jump, then another, then another. The distance is measured to the closest heel. Take the best jump of three (players find this fun, but don't let them do more than their three, as they will be quite sore the next day). It's interesting that the jump distance number (in feet) is similar to the one-step

At the Home Depot Center in Los Angeles, I watched the fitness testing practices for the under-19 and under-17 women's national teams. I wandered around the various stations and stopped at the standing triple jump. What caught my eye was the landing, especially the landing of the final jump. The girls basically could be divided into two distinct groups. One group landed with a good, wide base of support, with their knees nicely bent to absorb the shock of landing. The other group landed with a narrower base and very obviously knock-kneed.

One of the common mechanisms of an ACL injury is a stiff, erect landing with knock-knees. When one lands with a wide base, it is impossible to land erect; and it is tough for a knock-kneed landing to achieve that same wide base.

I have no data to support this next statement, but I'll say it anyway. If I were to see players landing knock-kneed in this standing triple jump, I would immediately put them on a prevention program (actually, I would include a prevention program for all girls middle school–age and older). I think those players are at an increased risk of an ACL injury. Of course, there will be players who land properly and tear their ACLs, just as there will be players who always land knock-kneed and never tear an ACL. However, due to the prevalence of this injury in female athletes, the preferred action is for coaches to put all girls on a prevention program.

vertical jump height (in inches). Watch players closely when they do this one. If they land with what some Europeans call "kissing knees" (knock-kneed), they may be at risk for an ACL injury. Landings should be with the feet apart and the knees over the feet, not knocking into each other.

Local muscle endurance. Actual, brute strength is less of a concern than is a muscle group's ability to keep working over time. The two most common tests are the 1-minute sit-up and 1-minute push-up. These test the endurance of the abdominals and the shoulders. These are done in pairs. For the sit-ups, the player lies with the knees bent at about 90 degrees, with the feet held firm by the partner. Start the clock, and see how many sit-ups the player can do in a minute. Record the results and swap players. The push-ups are started in the up position (younger women can do male or "female" push-ups; it doesn't matter—just be consistent). The partner lies in front with an arm extended and hand in a fist located on the ground under the sternum. Start the clock, and the partner counts the number of times the chest hits his fist. I know what you are thinking, and the answer is yes, players hate to do these. Only do one trial of each; high school girls should aim for totals in the upper 30s to 40s, 40s to 50s for boys.

Agility. The ability to change direction and position accurately is agility. It's one of those things we know when we see it. I think of Barry Sanders as the embodiment of agility. There are many tests of agility. Just pick one, and stick with it. Most players have fun doing agility tests.

A popular one is the 20-yard pro agility drill, made famous by the National Football League (NFL). Three lines are laid out on the field, parallel to each other and 5 yards apart. The player straddles the middle line. On the "go" command, the player moves to the right to touch the line, then all the way to the left to touch that line, and back to the center line. This test is simple, quick, and fun, but limited. Why? I've tested ninth-grade girls on this test, as well as the best collegiate women, and the differences between the two age groups are minimal. I don't think the test is long enough to discriminate between abilities and ages. Still, if you like this test, take the average of the two best of three runs. The time on this test will be pretty similar to a 40-yard dash.

Figure 2.7 is one example of a longer test, called the Illinois Agility Run. The player begins lying on her stomach, knees bent slightly (which keeps them from "digging in" for the start), and arms slightly off the ground. On the "go" command, she scrambles to her feet and follows the course. Do this three times, and take the average of the best two runs.

Another test is called the T-test. A course in the shape of a "T" is laid out on the ground. Each leg of the T is 10 yards long. Use cones at the start, at the intersection of the two lines, and at each end of the cross of the T. The player starts at the bottom of the T. On the "go" command, he sprints to the middle cone, shuffles to the right, sprints all the way to the left, shuffles back to the middle cone, then runs backward to the start. As always, do three trials and take the average of the two fastest.

Anaerobic capacity. Some people like to test for anaerobic capacity. I am not one of them anymore (I used to test for this), but two tests are typically used. One is a 300-meter sprint on a track—simple and straightforward. The other is a 300-meter shuttle. A corner flag is placed at the start, then every 10 meters out to 50 meters from

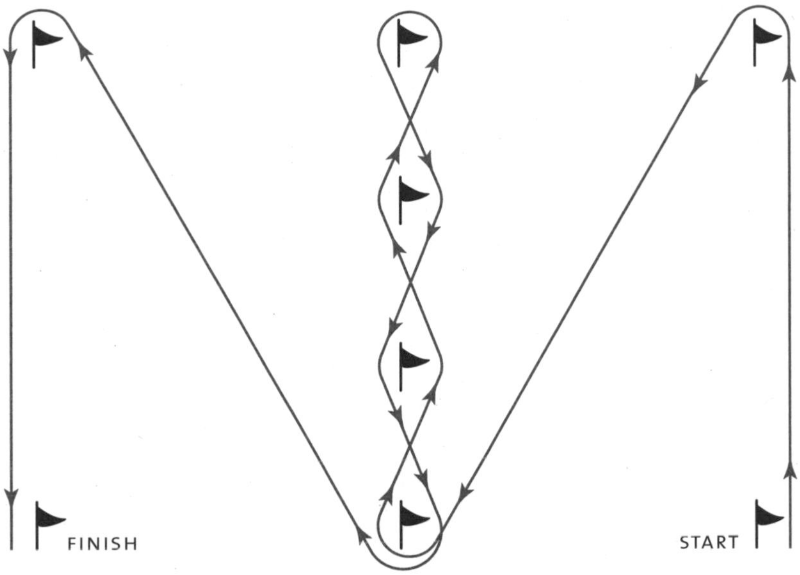

FIGURE 2.7

Illinois Agility Run

FINISH

START

10 YARD X 10 YARD BOX

the start flag. On the "go" command, the player runs to the first flag and around it, then back around the start flag, then out to the second flag, and so forth (he can start out going to the farthest flag first if he wants). The total distance is 300 meters. There are runs of different lengths with lots of changes of directions. So why don't I like these types of tests? Tell me when during soccer do players run like either test—45–70 seconds of solid, high-intensity running? I prefer to test for the specific aspects of fitness that fit the game, and this one doesn't. If you wish to use either test, only test once. Be ready for anything. I've seen more than one player lose his most recent meal after doing the 300-meter shuttle.

Endurance

Most people in the game consider endurance to be the most important fitness factor in soccer. There are five commonly used tests of endurance: two runs for time (1 or 2 miles) or distance (12-minute run) or either of two tests the kids call "beep" tests, which are administered using a commercial audiotape or compact disc.

1- or 2-mile run. This test is simple. On the track have the players run 1 or 2 miles as fast as possible (middle schoolers would do a mile,

While living in Cleveland in the mid-1980s, I got to know the coaches for the Cleveland Force Major Indoor Soccer League. The head coach, Timo Liekoski, and his chief assistant, Jay Hoffman, had an interesting philosophy about pro soccer players. They thought that every one of their players should be able to run 2 miles in 12 minutes simply because they were properly motivated professionals. So the 12-minute run in and of itself was not usable for him. However, if the players had done their training homework and were properly fit, they would be able to do that 2-mile run in 12 minutes again the next day. Sure enough, on the first day of fitness testing, the bulk of the players made the 2-mile run in 12 minutes. The next day was a different story: nowhere near the same number made the mark the second time around. Only those who had done their summer homework were able to do the 12-minute 2-mile run the second day.

high school and older players would do 2 miles). Some people split the difference and test a 1.5-mile run time. Do this in two groups, and have a partner record the time called out as each player finishes. High school boys should run 1.5 miles in around 8–9 minutes or less and girls in 10–12 minutes or less.

12-minute run. This was made famous in the late 1960s as a field predictor of vo_2 max and is still a great test for that purpose. Simply put, the players cover as much distance as possible in 12 minutes. A high school boy should be very close to 2 miles in 12 minutes (7–8 laps of a standard running track). High school girls should be able to run around 1.5 miles or a bit better (6–7 laps of that same track).

Beep tests. There are two primary "beep" tests currently in use. Each uses a 20-meter shuttle run. Two parallel lines are marked out 20 meters apart. The players run back and forth, paced by tones on an audiotape or compact disc. The pace of the runs gets gradually faster until the player is unable to keep pace with the tape, and then he is done. The farther one goes on the test, the better the endurance.

One is the continuous Leger test (the original test). On this tape, the pace is continuous. The players just keep running back and forth until they can't keep pace with the tape.

The other is called the Yo-Yo intermittent recovery run. This is like the Leger, except that it has a 10-second pause after each down-and-back 20-meter shuttle. (Administering this test takes a little practice, so never let the first time you do it be on your players. It is best to set the test up and try it out before putting your charges through it.) In this test the pace gradually increases until the player fails to keep pace on two runs. After the second failure, the player is asked to step off (this is usually not hard to see: when they are done, they are obviously done), and the total number of runs or the distance covered (number of runs x 40 meters) is recorded. Both beep tests take around 8–12 minutes to do unless some player has exceptional endurance.

I prefer the Yo-Yo beep test for a number of reasons. First, soccer is about recovery, and this format tests the player's ability to recover after moderate-intensity runs. Second, soccer is not a game of continuous running, like the track tests or the Leger version. Third, the published research shows the Yo-Yo test is a good predictor of match running performance for both players and referees.

My final reason dates back to an experience that I will attribute

Some important tips "from the trenches" from having run hundreds of players through the beep test:

1 Always use a boombox with fresh batteries so that the speed of tape playback is consistent. Use a battery-powered unit so there is no extension cord to trip over and stop the test. A compact disc is even better because a tape stretches out with usage.

2 Girls especially will cheer on their teammates. With all the cheering going on, it gets hard to hear the beeps, especially at the far turn. Players need to know that the runners have to hear the tape. Don't discourage cheering but have them stop when the beep is due. It really sounds odd with the on-and-off cheering.

3 When the test gets down to fewer and fewer runners, you can move them in closer to each other (and the boombox) so they support each other on each run. Don't allow players not being tested to pace players still running.

4 The test stops when the player can't keep up with the pace the second time. Some players will use their first failure for extra recovery; that is, they trot out a few steps, turn and return, and wait for the next repetition. Don't allow it. They must try on each run.

5 The player gets credit for starting that last run. So when the player is spent, encourage him to at least start one more as that one counts, even though he won't get very far.

6 Keep water nearby for each player. They have plenty of time for sips between runs.

7 Set up the course with cones so players run a straight line. The best way is to set up cones of alternating colors on the start and at turn lines. (April Heinrichs taught me that one.) That way, the player runs toward that orange cone or the yellow cone in front of her. You will be surprised how many players will make a diagonal run as they tire.

8 There are lots of instructions on the tape. Just rewind it back to "Now, get ready to start the test." Once you've done it or seen it, no reason to listen to all the instructions again. It is easy to learn.

9 Remind the players that the idea on this test is to run as a group. It does no one any real good to outrun their teammates on any individual run. Where you outrun your teammates is on the total distance covered.

10 Unless you happen to be on artificial turf, run this test in studs to avoid slipping at the turns.

to dumb luck. April Heinrichs had a national team camp in Florida one January and expanded the number of players to bring in some young talent to train with the "regulars." They all went through some of these fitness tests. At this camp, the players ran the continuous Leger test. About a week later, the younger players went to an under-19 camp in San Diego where they went through many of the same tests again under different supervision, only this time, they did the Yo-Yo intermittent recovery test, not the Leger test.

I managed to get the results for both tests. In Florida the two young goalkeepers finished in the middle of the under-19 group of field players, but in California the goalkeepers covered about 20–25% less distance than the same field players tested the week before. Intuitively, that makes sense. Do you really think goalkeepers have similar soccer-specific endurance as field players? That little series of events convinced me to use the intermittent recovery test exclusively.

A Resource You Should Have

Performance Conditioning, Inc., in Lincoln, Nebraska, publishes newsletters and specialized pamphlets on fitness for a number of different sports, soccer included, and a really good one is *A Guide to Soccer Field Testing* (I wrote parts of it, but I get no money out of the sales). There are lots of standards from folks other than me on things like the 1-, 1.5-, 2-mile, and 12-minute run, other sprints, and more. (See the Resources list at the end of this book for ordering information.)

When to Test

Now that you've decided to test your players, the typical question is when to test. Anson Dorrance tests his women on a reasonable schedule. Most seasons in the United States are quite short when compared with those of our European or South American friends. Typically, a team has a focused season—fall, for example. After the fall season is done, the players usually take some time off. Many teams test at the end of this off-season, sometime in January or February. Then, there is usually spring season (that is not the focused, important season). At the end of this spring season, test the team again. This serves two purposes: it shows the players how much they have improved over the spring, but more important, it serves as the level of fitness that the players must at least meet when they arrive at camp for the fall season, when they are tested again. The players have a goal (the spring tests) and have to train during the summer to maintain and improve their fitness. What happens if the players fail to duplicate or beat their spring tests? Well, Anson has this little group called The Breakfast Club . . . you get the idea, I am sure. Better to run during the summer than join that club.

Testing Results

Table 2.2 provides the average results of the various fitness tests for various age groups and levels of play. Check for the age and gender of interest to see some representative results.

Recommendations for a Fitness Testing Day

I base my test battery on experience, economy of time, and the nature of the game. Soccer is all about recovery, and I have described two tests of recovery: recovery from high-intensity running (7 x 30 meter sprints) and recovery from moderate-intensity running (Yo-Yo intermittent recovery shuttle). Soccer is also about power, so I do a vertical jump test. Finally, one thing that seems to separate soccer players from other athletes is agility. I do not favor doing multiple tests of the same factor, so I only recommend one test of leg power, one test of agility, and one test of endurance. I will be the first to agree that agility tests are fun, but do you get any more information with three tests than you would have gotten from one? Keep it short, keep it simple, and get the most information possible.

On a day of testing, here is how I organize the tests. You may change things around a bit to suit your circumstances. A good warm-up precedes the testing.

1 Divide the team in half. Half the players do the 7 x 30 sprints. The other half is split equally between the vertical jump and the agility test. Those doing the agility and vertical jump tests will finish first, so they then swap stations. After this group has done their two tests, those doing the 7 x 30 sprints should about be done (especially if you can double up the runners, as described above). Swap the runners with the others. The runners split between the agility and vertical jump tests, while those who have completed the agility and vertical jump now do the 7 x 30 sprints.

2 Redivide the players in half again. Half the players (usually those who did the 7 x 30s first (but that isn't a requirement) will do the Yo-Yo test, and the other half watch. When coaches get good at doing this test, they can usually watch and record results on 4–5 players at a time, leaving the other players free to encourage their teammates. Once the first group is done, the data is collected, and the second group does the test. All told, this period of

TABLE 2.2 Fitness Test Results

Classification	Speed (Meters/ Second)[a]	Vertical Jump (Inches)[b]	Pro Agility (Seconds)	Illinois Agility (Seconds)	300- Meter Shuttle	Intermittent Recovery (Meters)[c]
Girls[d]						
Under 12	5.65	16	5.85		76.26	528
Under 13	5.4	16	5.88	18.71	77.66	529
Under 14	5.68	18.5	5.45	19.11	75.64	586
Under 15	5.63	18	5.49	17.79	73.88	755
Under 16	5.6	18	5.34	18.62	75.81	625
Under 18	5.79	18.5	5.35	18.77	73.76	585
Boys[d]						
Under 12	5.26	18		18.62	80.22	723
Under 13	5.79	18		17.93	74.92	717
Under 14	6.10	20.5		17.62	71.78	1,043
Under 15	5.68	22.5		17.34	67.21	1,148
Under 16	5.54	22.5		17.68	70.78	938
Elite women						
College		20		16.83	67.37	1,216
Under 21	7.17	21		16.68	64.24	1,374
National	7.33	22		16.20	65.55	1,310
Elite men						
Under 17	7.78	26		15.73	63.47	1,401
Under 20	8.77	28		15.00	62.38	638[e]
Under 23	8.01	28		15.19	62.62	678[e]
National	8.45	27		15.33	60.24	857[e]

Source: This table represents a summary of data I have collected over the years. The youth data are from North Carolina Classic League teams in and around the Triangle.

a. The sprint speeds are in meters per second. This shows the increase in speed across levels of play better than reporting the results in elapsed time. For the youth teams, these speeds come from a hand-timed 200-yard sprint, where the players began from a standing start. For the elite players, the speeds are from electronic timing during the fastest 20-meter split of 7 x 30 meter sprints.

b. The vertical jump heights are all from a one-step approach to a two-foot takeoff. The results are rounded to the nearest half inch, as most people are likely to be accurate to half an inch. Most all results were obtained using a Vertec, which measures to the half inch.

When you look at table 2.2, take note of a couple things:

1 Notice that the intermittent recovery test (the beep test) results for the youth teams don't really change all that much with each older age group. Not much emphasis is being placed on endurance training in the youth programs.

2 Most players and parents would think that playing in the traveling program for their state would be good preparation for playing in college. The results for the oldest youth group versus the college (for women) or the elite men's under-20 team (whose player pool is largely the U.S. university program plus some Major League Soccer players) argue otherwise, though. There is quite a jump in performance, especially in endurance. For example, endurance in college women (1,216 meters) is over double that of the under-18 girls (585 meters). The traveling player who assumes he is physically prepared for college is in for a rude awakening when fall practice starts. Club training may be good for tactics and technique, but when it comes to fitness, most clubs do not prepare players physically for "the next level."

Notes to Table 2.2 (continued)

c. Most intermittent recovery shuttle tests were level 1, which starts slower and progresses more slowly than level 2, which is reserved for elite adult males. There is no correction factor to convert level 1 to level 2 results for easy comparisons. If elite adult males do level 1 of the test, the total duration could easily exceed 20 minutes, thus the faster test.

d. All youth data were obtained from Classic level (traveling) teams in North Carolina. All tests were done on grass with the players wearing their cleated shoes.

e. Level 2 intermittent recovery shuttle tests.

1 No matter what agility test is used, it will tear up the grass, so be careful where you set it up. The Illinois Agility Run is set up in a 10 x 10 yard box. To spread out the abuse on the grass, players can alternate the start/finish lines. You can also move the start/finish points to the opposite sides of the box, or you can simply rotate the flag setup by 90 degrees by remeasuring those flags up the middle. This only takes a minute or two, especially if you plan it out ahead of time.

2 At one point in the beep test players turn 180 degrees. I usually set this point up on the side (touch) line so it is out of the way. Don't put this turnaround on the field as the players will practically dig "starting blocks" in the dirt with each successive turn, and that will make for hazardous conditions on the field once practice starts.

3 The easiest setup for the 7 x 30s is along a touch line. Make sure you put cones to guide the players back to the starting line and for other players to avoid. Most electronic timers use some sort of photocell, and you don't want someone activating the timers during someone's run. Have the starting line maybe 1 yard before the timer beam. Some players dip their head or swing their arms very big when they start and can trigger the timers early.

4 Use the whole field. There is no need to have the test stations on top of each other.

5 Be sensitive to the field conditions before you start and consider what you will leave afterward for either the next team or the groundskeeper.

testing can be done in 1.5 hours once you get good at organizing the session.

ERGOGENIC AIDS

If you follow international soccer, you might remember when FIFA announced that the Netherlands's Edgar Davids and Portuguese national team captain Fernando Couto were among eight players in the Italian Serie A league who tested positive for the steroid nandrolone and were suspended from international play. Davids's Dutch teammate Frank de Boer was also under investigation. Positive tests for nandrolone are almost epidemic and routinely make front-page news.

Typically, players claim innocence, insisting someone gave them a tainted supplement. The suspension is appealed, but they end up serving the suspension. *No* sport governing body accepts ignorance

College, national, and international competitive events all conduct announced and random testing for doping agents. The list is long, and it contains items that some believe need not be tested for. FIFA defines doping as "any attempt either by a player, or at the instigation of another person such as a manager, coach, trainer, doctor, physiotherapist or masseur, to enhance mental and physical performance unphysiologically or to treat ailments or injury—when such treatment is medically unjustified—for the sole purpose of taking part in a competition." The goals of doping control are laudable:

• To uphold and preserve the ethics of the game
• To safeguard the physical health and mental integrity of the player
• To ensure that all competitors have an equal chance

FIFA first conducted drug testing in 1966, but over the past 10–12 years it has shifted into high gear. Since 1994, FIFA has conducted over 3,000 tests at the finals competitions of the world championships and Olym-pics (as of 2005). During that time, FIFA has found a total of three positive tests, and only one of those was for an anabolic steroid. This is a 0.09% incidence of positive tests. If one looks at all doping control tests for soccer conducted by the International Olympic Committee laboratories, there have been a total of 88 positive samples out of nearly 21,000 tests, and 75% of those positive tests were for recreational drugs (marijuana and cocaine). In general, team sports have nowhere near the use of banned substances that plagues individual sports like weight lifting, running, cross-country skiing, cycling, and others. Those sports have a single particular aspect of fitness that can be manipulated by doping and improve the athlete's chance of success. Team sports don't seem to have a single factor of fitness that can be manipulated by drugs and impact the outcome of a match. That and the sport's governing bodies have exercised due diligence in their fight against doping.

as an excuse: you took it, you tested positive, you should've known, you are suspended. The WADA (World Anti-Doping Agency) wants all first positive tests to lead to a lengthy suspension of 1–2 years.

Just what is nandrolone? It's a prescription anabolic-androgenic steroid that was popular among strength athletes as far back as the 1970s due to its effectiveness in producing muscle growth and speeding recovery with minimal side effects. Unlike testosterone, this synthetic steroid has strong anabolic properties (muscle building), but only moderate androgenic properties (secondary male sex characteristics).

Nandrolone does have legitimate medical uses in treating anemia or selected kidney disorders. Nandrolone also increases hemoglobin and red blood cell mass, making it popular with some endurance athletes.

The use of nandrolone declined quickly when it was added to the drug-testing list in 1975. Even in incredibly small amounts, nandrolone can be detected, and it stays in the body for a very long period of time. A urine sample may be positive for 60 days or more after the last dose. That's why athletes taking nandrolone get caught in random drug tests.

Nandrolone is produced in small amounts by the body. Laboratories accredited by the International Olympic Committee (IOC) have reported over 300 positive tests for nandrolone in a variety of sports. The labs say the amounts detected far exceed that produced naturally. Nandrolone and its metabolites are tested in the laboratory by a method called gas chromatography/mass spectroscopy, and the test is accurate over 99% of the time. The false positive rate is less than 1 in 10,000 tests.

If nandrolone is on the banned list and is so easily detected, isn't it odd that athletes continue to test positive for nandrolone? Are athletes consciously testing their fates with this drug in the name of greater glory? Something else must be going on.

This increase could be explained by newer "nutritional supplements" that can be purchased over the counter in many stores and over the Internet. These supplements are termed "prohormones." A prohormone is any steroid-like substance that remotely resembles testosterone and might serve as a building block for testosterone. Prohormones also refer to any steroid-like substance that might exert an anabolic and/or androgenic action similar to testosterone or one of its synthetic derivatives. The public's awareness of these substances was raised with androstenedione, used by Mark McGuire, and androstenediol.

When the first of these prohormones was released, the scientific community found that these substances converted mostly to the female hormone estrogen and not into testosterone. In men, high levels of estrogen relative to testosterone have been associated with a variety of abnormalities, including heart disease, prostate problems, and breast development. So in response to these potential health problems the supplement industry came up with the so-called 19-nor prohormones.

For you organic chemists, the modified prohormones androstenedione and androstenediol lack a carbon group at position number 19 on the steroid backbone. At best, they are distant cousins of testosterone, but more closely resemble nandrolone, also a 19-nor substance. However, unlike the nonprescription 19-nors, nandrolone is only available with a prescription because it is a proven anabolic steroid.

In fact, both 19-norandrostenedione and 19-norandrostenediol (two popular over-the-counter 19-nor prohormones) so closely resemble nandrolone in structure that they are either identified in the body as nandrolone or can actually be converted into nandrolone once in the system.

Herein lies the problem for athletes. To athletes wanting more muscle mass, 19-nors look like a dream—essentially an over-the-counter nandrolone, producing muscle mass without a prescription. However, athletes in competitions where drug testing is performed are asking to get caught.

So, are athletes coming up positive because they are taking a "supplement," or are they actually taking the banned substance nandrolone? What difference does it make? Both they and their teams suffer.

The bottom line is this: no professional and Olympic athlete should take these supplements because their urine will test positive for nandrolone in as little as 3 days and for as long as 60 or more days. Here is a quotation from a website selling these products: "The product has a very long half life and should be discontinued at least 60 days prior to being drug tested."

The moral of the story: stay informed. Read labels and know what you are taking in supplement form. I even saw an Internet company whose creatine monohydrate is boosted with a 19-nor additive. Just because something is sold over the counter or by mail order and labeled as "natural" does not mean it is safe to use—and most of all it could lead to a positive drug test.

Creatine Use in Soccer

Many soccer players and coaches are asking questions about the use of creatine for improving performance. There are reports of professional players in England, Brazil, Argentina, and more using creatine in order to train harder. There are probably many more. There is little talk of using creatine for games. A summary of creatine use (and other supplements) written by the U.S. Olympic Committee (USOC) is available on request from the USOC Sport Science and Technology Department or at <http://www.usoc.org/12694.htm>.

Creatine is naturally found in the body and is also in the diet (from meat and fish). Its main use is the transfer of energy in cells. The thought is that a greater intake of creatine will help in the rapid turn-over of energy during exercise. The use of creatine is not banned by the USOC, IOC, NCAA, or FIFA, but sport organizations are looking closely at this issue, and no governing body endorses its use. NCAA Division I universities are prohibited from supplying creatine to athletes.

High-intensity, intermittent exercise like soccer needs a rapid transfer of energy, and creatine plays a critical role in energy trans-fer. Many studies have shown that high-intensity work and recovery after and between bouts of high-intensity work can be improved with creatine supplementation. Most of these studies use weight training or limited repeats of sprinting in a laboratory. Low-intensity, long-duration exercise requires a steady production of energy at a slow rate. Creatine does not improve aerobic (cycling or running) perfor-mance. Recovery from high-intensity exercise is enhanced with cre-atine supplementation. If athletes recover faster, then perhaps they can begin the next exercise session sooner, or they can train at a higher intensity. Either method increases the quality of training. This has not been studied systematically, yet the use of creatine as a train-ing aid (as opposed to a performance aid on "game day") has been practiced in many sports.

Most research about creatine is laboratory-based and has little ap-plication to any playing field. Creatine has been shown to improve performance in high-intensity exercise (e.g., weight lifting, sprinting), but those exercise sessions were very short (e.g., six 60-meter sprints), which is far below what soccer training or competition entails. *There are no data to suggest that creatine supplementation will improve per-formance for soccer players during a match*, but there are some reports that creatine does improve some tests of soccer performance that are of very short duration, similar to the repeated sprint tests so often reported. Creatine may help lead to faster recovery, which may allow the player to go through higher-quality training, which could lead to improved fitness and game performance. However, remember that the current work on creatine is largely for very high-intensity, short-duration exercises like weight lifting and sprinting and not on lower-intensity, longer-duration exercises like soccer. You can find a more detailed report on creatine and soccer (by me) at the Gatorade Sports Science Institute (<www.gssiweb.com>).

The fact is we need to know more about creatine use in soccer:

1 Creatine does not work in everybody. Some people are called "nonresponders," and there is no way to determine who will or will not respond.

2 Some athletes complain of muscle and gastrointestinal cramping, but there is little scientific evidence in this area.

3 When you take a supplement, your own body's production of that substance can be reduced, reducing the energy-enhancing effects of creatine.

4 You must be concerned with the purity with any dietary supplements. Control of over-the-counter commercial supplements is not very rigid. Appeals by athletes who tested positive after taking a supplement that contained a substance banned by the NCAA, USOC, FIFA, or IOC are routinely denied. Some athletes will even keep a pill or two from a bottle, just in case they test positive and need to retest the batch they had. No court of appeal or opinion would believe that those pills were from that same batch.

5 Finally, there is the concern about side effects. Rapid weight gain is the most common side effect. Few women use it for this reason, and many men elect not to use creatine for the same reason The weight gain can be dramatic: 10 pounds in a week or two is not unusual. There also are individual reports about the effect of high doses of creatine on the kidneys, but there are no long-term studies that might tell us about potential side effects of chronic use. All the published reports on potential clinical issues regarding creatine are dated before the year 2000, with no new reports since then. Ongoing, unpublished research says the use of creatine may lead to the development of chronic compartment syndromes in the legs.

Anabolic/Androgenic Steroids

Whenever the topic of drugs and sports comes up, anabolic steroids are usually the first drug discussed. While the taking of steroids is not a common practice in soccer (in spite of the recent positive test on Christophe Dugarry of the French national team), they are used in high schools, and not just for sports. Please be aware that the steroids someone gets injected into a joint or takes for asthma are totally different from anabolic steroids. It is important to say at the start that the use of anabolic/androgenic steroids is banned by virtually every federation that sponsors international competition. The IOC, FIFA, and NCAA all outlaw their use.

Anabolic/androgenic steroids are artificial mimics of testosterone and have limited, but important, clinical uses. They may be prescribed as replacement therapy for a patient who has had surgical or traumatic removal of the testicles. They may also be prescribed for muscle-wasting diseases, in an attempt to minimize the loss of muscle mass, and some anemias. The "anabolic" in the name relates to the steroid's ability to build tissue, while "androgenic" refers to secondary sex characteristics. There are many types of steroids on the market with varying degrees of anabolic and androgenic properties.

These drugs were developed in the 1940s, but the widespread use of steroids began in the early 1960s in the weight training community because of the increase in muscle mass. They have since spread to other sports where muscle mass, strength, and high power output are important. Moreover, their use has spread beyond sports to nonathletes, who use steroids to get big, just for the aesthetics; high school boys are taking steroids to impress girls. Women athletes have been known to use steroids, but the side effects of masculinizing secondary sex characteristics are a real problem.

The question that has always been asked is, "Do they work?"—and the answer is a qualified "yes." If the drugs are taken in therapeutic doses, the potential effects are slight. To have a significant effect, however, the dosage needs to be similar to the testosterone surge during puberty, and that dose is a lot higher than therapeutic levels. Steroid users have plenty of experience with drug choices, administration scheduling, and avoiding detection. Steroids seem to have the most benefit in experienced weight lifters. Inexperienced lifters seem to have little if any response to steroids. So, the effectiveness of ste-

Cardiovascular disease is a well-known complication of steroid abuse. If you were ever able to go "backstage" at the NFL combine, where potential players are paraded around in their shorts, you will see that some team reps have a check-off for acne. Why acne? Remember that anabolic steroids sort of mimic puberty with a rush of testosterone-like hormones—and acne hits boys the hardest during puberty. So a big, 22-year-old college football player with a substantial case of acne just might be taking steroids, and that is a no-no in the NFL.

So, just how extensive are the side effects of anabolic steroids? The list is pretty extensive. Many of these are reversed once steroids are discontinued.

Liver
  Abnormal liver enzymes
  Blood-filled cysts
  Benign tumors
  Malignant tumors
Male reproductive system
  Reduced system of reproductive hormones
  Reduced sperm production
  Testicular atrophy
  Breast formation

Female reproductive system
  Reduction in circulating sex hormones
  Menstrual irregularities
  Masculinization of the female (facial hair, deepening voice, male pattern baldness, breast atrophy, clitoral hypertrophy)
Cardiovascular system
  Lipid profile changes to that similar to people with heart disease
  Elevated total cholesterol and some increase in LDL (low-density lipoprotein) cholesterol
  Drastically reduced HDL (high-density lipoprotein) cholesterol, well below normal levels
  Possible elevation of blood pressure
Psychological effects
  Increased aggressiveness ("'roid rage")
  Sleep disorders
  Anxiety and paranoia
  Some users have reported hallucinations
  Withdrawal symptoms
Other side effects
  Altered thyroid function
  Some suggestion of altered immune function
  Decreased glucose tolerance and increased insulin resistance (like type II diabetes)

roids depends on all the variables of dosage and the experiences of the user.

The effects of steroids are wide-ranging. Testosterone is associated with increasing masculinity, male sexual maturity, aggression, and sex drive, and some of these characteristics are prized in selected sports. Anabolic steroids have similar effects even in women, resulting in the growth of body hair, deepening of the voice, and more.

Metabolic reworking of excess testosterone also can lead to some increases in estrogen in men to the extent that men develop breast tissue. Beyond this, replacement of natural testosterone with a drug can lead the testicles to function at a lower level and shrink. Further, damage to the liver (blood-filled cysts), heart (coronary heart disease), and blood vessels (stroke), and even cancer, have been linked to long-term steroid use. A cousin's daughter once commented on these two "beautiful" guys who lived across the street, but strangely each had suffered a stroke before his twenty-first birthday. One even hears about early steroid users having open heart surgery at very young ages.

There has been a lot of press lately on the number of positive tests for nandrolone in people who have long histories of clean tests (as in Dugarry's case). As mentioned, the urine tests for steroids are so sensitive that extremely small amounts can be detected, and there is a question about whether over-the-counter supplements have minute amounts of nandrolone that lead to all these positive tests. The IOC so far has turned a deaf ear to athletes who have tested positive, saying it is the athlete's responsibility to know what is in any supplement he or she is taking. These drugs are not to be messed with, and they certainly have no place in soccer.

"Andro" and Testosterone: Why It's So Hard to Say a Supplement Works

In the search for more "natural" anabolic support, athletes have been turning to testosterone precursors to increase naturally occurring testosterone (or to "designer" steroids — as in the BALCO case). If more of the precursors are available, then perhaps more testosterone will be around and then give the anabolic effects of increased testosterone. The most visible of these products is androstenedione ("andro") that practically became a household word when it was disclosed that Mark McGwire was taking this supplement during his record-breaking home run season of 1998.

Androstenedione is a precursor to testosterone and is produced by the adrenal glands and the gonads. It is converted to testosterone and estrogen, thus it is thought that increasing androstenedione may result in an increase in both testosterone and estrogen. One unit of androstenedione does not lead to one unit of testosterone, so large amounts of the precursor must be consumed. When reading a study of any precursor supplement, the dosage and dosing schedule must be considered. In many projects, the ingested amount is pretty low.

There are other precursors available over the counter at nutrition stores and in magazine ads. For example, androstenediol and DHEA (dehydroepiandrosterone) also convert to testosterone. The 19-nor products (19-norandrostenedione and 19-norandrostenediol) both are metabolized to nandrolone (a banned substance) and eventually testosterone. These products are significant because most of the highly publicized positive drug tests reported by the NCAA and other sporting organizations over the past two years have been due to supplements, specifically these 19-norandro products.

People use androstenedione because of an early report on two women whose testosterone levels tripled in response to treatment. What the makers don't tell you is that their testosterone returned to normal in only a couple of hours. This simple research paper is the basis for all the advertising claims supporting androstenedione. Five recent research studies only confuse the issue because two showed increases in testosterone, while three failed to show any increase. A look at why the supplement literature is so confusing and difficult to interpret might be educational for players and parents alike.

1 Androstenedione and DHEA were compared with a placebo. Strength-training subjects ingested 100 milligrams a day for 12 weeks. Blood, body composition, and performance variables were assessed before, during, and after the study. While there were small increases in strength and lean mass in the experimental groups, the differences were not statistically different from the placebo group (M. Brian Wallace et al., *Medicine and Science in Sports and Exercise*, 1999).

2 Acute (i.e., single dose) and long-term responses to androstenedione ingestion (300 milligrams a day) were compared. Blood (testosterone, estrogen, lipids), muscle cell area, body composition, and strength were studied in male strength-training novices. While acute ingestion led to increases in serum androstenedione, no changes were seen in testosterone. Chronic use was the same, yet estrogen was increased significantly. Neither strength increases nor muscle cell changes were different between groups. HDL (high-density lipoproteins—the good cholesterol)

dropped over the 8-week project in the andro group only, which is not good (Douglas S. King et al., *Journal of the American Medical Association*, 1999).

3 An acute response to a 200-milligram dose showed elevated testosterone in 90 minutes (T. N. Ziegenfuss et al., *Canadian Journal of Applied Physiology*, 2002).

4 In another project, subjects ingested 200 milligrams a day of androstenedione (vs. placebo) for 2 days, and blood was sampled for 3 days total. Exercise increased testosterone, with no difference between the andro group and placebo group. However, androstenedione did increase circulating estrogen (C. S. Ballantyne et al., *Canadian Journal of Applied Physiology*, 2000).

5 Finally, subjects were randomized to 100 milligrams a day, 300 milligrams a day of androstenedione or placebo groups for a week. Blood was sampled many times over the week. On day 7, testosterone was elevated in the high-dose group, while estradiol was elevated in both experimental groups (G. A. Brown et al., *Hormone and Metabolic Research*, 2004).

Confused? You should be. Looks like the scientific literature can't come to a decision on androstenedione. Here is where it starts to gets really confusing. Changes in blood levels of any hormone can be due to increased production, decreased elimination of the hormone, or a change in how tissues use the hormone. None of these studies talked about the turnover of the hormones other than to point out that these compounds have a very short life (minutes to hours). Also, is the "elevated" group truly elevated, or was the control group low to begin with? This opens the door to the question of nonresponders: the subject with normal levels of a variable, who shows little or no response. If the subject is low on the variable of interest, then any elevation might be significant. In the studies that show some effect of androstenedione, the testosterone levels in one study were 25% below those of another. In another, the only group that showed a significant increase in testosterone was the 300 milligrams per day group. Their initial levels were over 40% below those reported by others, and their peak levels were the same. Therefore, the question of the effectiveness of androstenedione seems to depend on the initial level of testosterone. And don't forget that the first report was on two women.

If all that didn't give you a headache, this might. There are at least five other factors to be considered when interpreting supplement research:

1 Anabolic steroids are most effective in experienced weight lifters; therefore, the experience of the subjects in weight training should be considered. Novice subjects might be expected to gain strength from beginning a weight-training program, and any possible additive effects of a supplement might be lost in the initial gain in strength.

2 The general feeling on strength gain is that initial gains in strength are due to increased recruitment of more muscle cells. Later gains in strength are from an increase in muscle mass. The time it takes for a subject to add hypertrophy to recruitment is quite variable from one person to the next. Thus, the length of any training study should be questioned. An 8-week study might be too brief to realize any real effects on muscle mass.

3 Aging has well-known effects on skeletal muscle and hormones. So, the age of subjects must be known when conclusions are drawn.

4 How were the hormones analyzed? Androstenedione has a very short life and can be rapidly incorporated into testosterone. Peak levels of testosterone from androstenedione ingestion occur quickly and last only a short time. Blood sampling has to be timed to find the peak response. Urine sampling might be the better method for such brief changes in testosterone (can you imagine weeks of 24-hour urine collection?)

5 Consider the ingestion schedule (and its interaction with the detection schedule). Would a single or twice per day dosing schedule be sufficient to chronically raise testosterone levels to have any real influence on muscle, when the high levels of testosterone are around only for a short time? Plus, consider the length of time the subjects ingested the andro. It is difficult to come up with a schedule when the duration of andro use was only one dose, 2 days, 1 week, 8 weeks, or 3 months.

Other concerns are the decrease in HDL-cholesterol and the consistent finding of increased estrogen. Low HDL-cholesterol is a known risk of heart disease. Elevated estrogen is a factor in gynecomastia (breast development in men), cardiovascular disease, and breast cancer. Plus, studies have shown that elevated androstenedione is linked to prostate and pancreatic cancer.

On closer scrutiny, it appears that androstenedione is only effective at bringing testosterone levels in men with low initial levels up to the levels seen in men with normal testosterone. Plus, there may be health consequences to long-term use that have yet to be proven.

From a practical standpoint, there has been a flood of positive drug tests for nandrolone across nearly all sports, not just for those normally associated with steroid abuse. Any athlete who is likely to be drug-tested needs to know that he or she may well test positive for steroids from these supplements. Ignorance is not an acceptable defense. Supplements are not subjected to the same Food and Drug Administration (FDA) regulations as prescription drugs, and makers are not required to list amounts of all ingredients on the labels. To avoid testing positive, all athletes should check with their institution and/or sports authority before taking any supplement.

The Next "Creatine"?

The best way to improve performance is to train properly and put the best fuel in the tank. Yet athletes continue to look for the next magic bullet while ignoring their basic nutrition. One new and one old supplement are making waves.

Ribose is a natural substance like creatine, and there are suggestions that ribose might improve athletic performance. Ribose is a five-carbon sugar that is involved with our main energy molecule, ATP. The theory is that by ingesting ribose one could replenish and store more ATP, which means more energy. You can find ribose in ripe fruits and vegetables; it was first reported to improve oxygen delivery in people with coronary heart disease. One manufacturer says that energy levels after high-intensity exercise can be restored in hours instead of days. The typical dose starts at 2.2 grams per day, progressing to 20–30 grams per day, but doses of up to 60 grams per day seem to be well tolerated. Theoretically, ribose supplementation might have some merit; however, there is no evidence to support its use. Why did it work in heart patients? Maybe because they had more to gain. The normal athlete does not appear to need any help on this level. Besides, it costs about a dollar per 2-gram dose. Spend the money on fresh food, not an unproven supplement.

Ephedrine is not a new stimulant. It was available for years at service station counters and was an ingredient in some over-the-counter weight-loss products. Ephedrine sales in 1999 were over $1 billion, but dollar volume did not equate with safety. This "amphetamine-like" compound stimulates the heart and nervous system and has been linked to several deaths. Ephedrine has been in the news a great deal. For example, ephedrine was part of the supplement cocktail that got Maradona kicked out of the 1994 World Cup. *Sports Illustrated* did a story in February 1998 on the use of an ephedrine (pseudoephedrine) in the National Hockey League. And ephedrine was mentioned in the investigations into the deaths of a couple of football players who were taking it when they died from heatstroke. The NFL, the NCAA, and the IOC (FIFA follows IOC rules) have all banned it. The NCAA reports that 4% of student athletes report having used ephedrine. The FDA has reported around 1,400 "events," with 80 deaths, associated with ephedrine. Heart attacks, strokes, and seizures are potential side effects. Read those labels.

Athletes seem to take ephedrine for one of two reasons. First is the stimulant effect. Athletes feel like they can train longer and harder. Second is the weight-loss effect. The stimulant features elevate the metabolic rate and burn calories, reducing weight. So far, no peer-reviewed journal articles have ever shown that ephedrine is effective at any level of sports performance.

There are dozens upon dozens of natural, herbal, and who-knows-what supplements one can get at a store, from a friend, and over the Internet. A discussion of all sports supplements is a book unto itself.

There are proven methods to improve performance—work hard and eat right. Nutritional modification has been shown over and over to improve performance, and it is a whole lot healthier. Make the right choices in the store, restaurant, and home. Supplements are a risk. As my friend Ron Maughan says, "If it works, it's probably banned. If it isn't banned, it probably doesn't work." There is a lot of truth in that statement.

Dr. Ron Maughan of Loughborough University in the United Kingdom is one of the most prolific researchers in nutritional supplements and sports performance. Here is an incomplete list of supplements he has investigated. These are most effective at emptying your wallet, not improving performance. Why is this list incomplete? Because tomorrow someone will come up with something new or make a claim about something old.

Acetylglutamine
Anabolic amino acids
Androstenedione
Antioxidants
Arginine
Ascorbic acid
Aspartate
Astragalus
Bee pollen
Bicarbonate
Bitter orange (Citrus aurantia)
Boron
Branched chain amino acids
Caffeine
Calcium
Carnitine
Chlorella

Choline
Chondroitin
Chromium
Chrysin
Coenzyme Q10
Colostrum
Cordyceps
Creatine
Echinacea
Eicosapentaenoic acid (EPA)
Energy bars
Essential amino acids
Essential fatty acids
Gamma-oryzanol
Ginkgo biloba
Ginseng
Glucosamine
Glutamine
Glycerol
Guarana
Hornet juice
Hydrolyzed proteins
Hydroxycitrate
Hydroxymethylbutyrate (HMB)
Inosine
Iron
Leucine
Lysine
Magnesium
Medium chain triglycerides
Melatonin

Methylsulphonylmethane (MSM)
Multivitamins
Mummio
Ornithine
Ornithine alpha-ketoglutarate
Phenylalanine
Phosphate
Protein
Protein hydrolysates
Pycnogenol
Pyruvate
Ribose
Royal jelly
S-adenosylmethionine (SAME)
Saw palmetto
Selenium
Smilax
Spirulina
Sports drinks
Taurine
Terrestris
Tribulus
Tryptophan
Tyrosine
Ubiquinone
Vanadium
Vitamin C
Vitamin E
Whey protein
Yohimbine
Zinc

Soccer is played in nearly every possible environment—from Antarctica to the African deserts. Some games at the World Cups in the United States (the men's tournament in 1994 and the women's in 1999 and 2003) and Spain (1982) were contested in oppressive heat (greater than 100 degrees Fahrenheit). In Mexico (1986), some games were played at altitude (greater than 7,000 feet), with heat and polluted air. In Korea (2002), the humidity (up to 85% and higher) was extremely challenging. Qualifying matches and professional league games in northern Europe can be played in cold weather. There are fields in Norway above the Arctic Circle. The sheer size of the United States means there are many different conditions possible, especially for the traveling team that participates around the country. That team from Vermont playing a spring tournament in Houston is in for a surprise. The summer USA Cup in Blaine, Minnesota, has been played in oppressive heat and humidity. Depending on the time of year and locale, the soccer player may have to play in any of these conditions.

Heat and Humidity

The environmental conditions that most soccer players will experience and should be of most concern to the coach, players, parents, and medical personnel are heat and humidity.

The problem of heat. Body temperature is a delicate balance of heat production and heat loss. Normal body temperature varies around 99 degrees Fahrenheit. Humans exist fairly close to our thermal boiling point; that means, our body temperature is closer to the high temperatures that can cause problems, but a greater temperature difference exists between our body temperature and dangerously cold levels

This can be a real problem during exercise. When we exercise, our body temperature rises, and without ways to lose heat, we would boil over very quickly. However, our system is quite adept at keeping our temperature from rising too high.

Where does our body temperature come from? Our bodies are always operating, even when we are at our lowest energy output. Much of the energy expended at rest is used to move electrolytes from the inside of cells to the outside and vice versa. Sodium is mostly outside the cell, and potassium is mostly inside the cell. When these end up in the other compartment, the cell tries to put them back where they are supposed to be. Energy is needed to operate this exchange pump. So the body breaks down ATP to ADP plus energy. Remember that at no time is all the energy harvested; some is used for work, and the rest is released as heat. Add up all the cells exchanging sodium and potassium and all the energy not used for this work that ends up as heat; this is the origin of our normal body temperature of 98.6 degrees Fahrenheit (37 degrees Celsius).

During exercise, those working muscles now break down much more ATP. The energy in each molecule is either used to power muscle contraction or released as heat. Add this to the basal temperature, and the overall body temperature rises above resting temperature. Now the body must get rid of the excess heat to avoid overheating. The body has a number of ways to do this:

- *Radiation*: This is probably the hardest for people to understand. Radiant energy waves move from the higher heat source to the lower source. An easily understood example is snow melting on a sunny, though below freezing, day. The snow melts as the radiant heat from the sun moves to the colder surface of the snow.
- *Conduction*: Ever put your hand on a cool surface and then notice that the cool surface gradually warms up? This is conduction. Heat moves downhill from the direct contact of the warm surface of the hand to the cool surface. Think of being sprayed with water, jumping into a pool, or draping a cold towel over the head—you cool off. Obviously, swimmers benefit from conductive heat transfer.
- *Convection*: If a cool breeze blows over the skin, heat is lost from the warm body to the cooler molecules of air. You are exposed to convective heat loss when you stand in front of a fan or air conditioner. Cyclists benefit from convective heat transfer.
- *Evaporation*: This is the most important method of heat loss during exercise. When the core temperature rises from all the heat produced by muscle contraction, cells transfer this heat to the blood. When the warm blood is transported back to the heart, it then passes over the body's thermostat (in the brain) called the hypothalamus. When the hypothalamus senses a rise in temperature, it sends out a signal to the blood vessels of the skin to dilate. Blood then is diverted to the cooler skin, and sweat is produced, which

moves to the surface. The actual loss of temperature is the result of this sweat evaporating to the environment. Dripping sweat is not heat loss—evaporating sweat is heat loss. Anything that hampers evaporation will make it more difficult for the body to lose heat.

The evaporation (not the production) of sweat is the actual transfer of heat. For each milliliter of water evaporated there is a loss of 0.6 kilocalories of heat energy. A casual athlete might lose up to 1 liter an hour of sweat, but the highly competitive athlete might lose up to 2 liters an hour of sweat, meaning there is the opportunity for extensive heat loss. Therefore, it is important to ensure that the barriers to evaporation (e.g., clothing, humidity) are minimal.

The American College of Sports Medicine (ACSM) has proposed limits on exercise and competition based on the radiant heat, humidity, and ambient temperature measured as the wet bulb globe temperature (WBGT). The formula is:

WBGT = (0.1 x ambient temp) + (0.2 x black globe temp) + (0.7 x wet bulb temp)

where "ambient temp" is the environmental temperature measured with a standard exterior thermometer; "black globe temp" is the temperature measured by a standard exterior thermometer inside a black, metal globe (for radiant temperature); and "wet bulb temp" is the temperature measured by a standard exterior thermometer with one end of a cotton wick over the mercury reservoir (the measuring tip) and the other end in water (for humidity).

It is easily seen that WBGT is heavily influenced by humidity (the 0.7), while ambient and radiant temperatures are less important (the 0.1 and 0.2, respectively). Thus, in the absence of a device to measure WBGT (either homemade or purchased—and these devices aren't cheap), humidity is a prime concern for athletes and should be known by attending medical personnel. The ACSM has recommended that sports participation be suspended if the WBGT exceeds 82 degrees. However, suspension may not be possible when mass-participation events (e.g., marathons) or spectator events (world championships, the Olympics, etc.) are scheduled far in advance due to time and economic constraints. Therefore, the medical staff of such an event must be prepared to treat heat illnesses.

In training, monitoring heart rate is sometimes used as a measure of exercise intensity. Remember that heart rate is affected by external temperature. Heart rate training zones are valid only for training at external temperatures between 15 and 25 degrees Celsius (roughly 60–75 degrees Fahrenheit), so players should be adapted for training in more extreme environmental temperatures. At high temperatures, heart rates are higher, and the same level of work feels harder, particularly if the high temperatures are associated with dehydration due to sweating. This heart rate "drift" differs significantly among individuals. Therefore, when training at high temperatures, be aware that the heart rate at any exercise level will be higher and the player's "perception" of training intensity will be higher. Adequate fluid replenishment during training is essential to avoid excessive increases of heart rate and impairment of training quality.

Heat Injury

Medical problems due to heat and humidity can run the spectrum of mild to fatal. Every physician who cares for athletes, as well as every coach, has to be aware of heat problems, their signs and symptoms, and initial treatment regardless of the level of athlete they deal with. Heat injury is probably the main concern of athletic trainers during summer football, soccer, and cross-country training.

"Heat cramps" is considered by many a misnomer. Many people have thought that imbalances of water and electrolytes (mostly sodium) were the cause of heat cramps. This has never been proven conclusively. Muscle cramps can occur at rest or during exercise, and seemingly successful treatment of exertional cramps with fluid and electrolyte therapy may simply be coincident with rest. Regardless, cramping requires some treatment: passive stretching, massage, or both by a trainer or physical therapist, combined with oral rehydration, preferably with sports beverages containing replacement electrolytes. Application of ice is often beneficial as well. Some individuals may respond better to an infusion of intravenous saline (normal saline or Lactated Ringers are the fluids physicians choose).

Heat exhaustion is a more serious condition, and left untreated, it may lead to heatstroke. Heat exhaustion is characterized by irritability, light-headedness, nausea (with or without vomiting), and generalized weakness. The player might have a rapid heart rate, low blood pressure, "goose bumps" (called piloerection), profuse sweating, and reduced urinary output. The core temperature is high but is less than 105 degrees Fahrenheit. Heat exhaustion is thought to be the result of dehydration and the resultant loss of blood volume (just where do you think the water for sweat comes from?). Electrolyte loss, particularly sodium, is also a contributing factor. Treatment for heat exhaustion requires rapid cooling in an attempt to reduce the core temperature to 102 degrees or less. Remove the player to a cool environment and spray him or her with cool or lukewarm water to help speed evaporation and conductive heat loss. A fan helps by adding convective heat loss. Oral rehydration is the preferred method of fluid replacement. However, the player who has severe nausea or vomiting may need intravenous fluids. In this situation, normal saline or Lactated Ringer's solutions are again the intravenous fluids chosen by the doctor.

Heatstroke is a medical emergency requiring immediate care. Rectal temperature is very high, 105 degrees Fahrenheit (41.8 degrees Celsius) or greater. Heatstroke is a global collapse of the body's means of heat loss. The reduction in blood volume and constriction of blood vessels at and near the skin (peripheral vasoconstriction) impair the body's ability to transfer heat to the environment. Signs and symptoms of exertional heatstroke include hypotension, fast heart rate (tachycardia), reduced urine output, vomiting, and diarrhea. The athlete may go into shock, which can lead to kidney failure. Disorientation and delirium are common, and there may even be bleeding into the brain; seizure activity and coma have been reported. Other organ systems can fail as well, including the hematologic system, liver, muscles (as rhabdomyolysis), lungs, and/or myocardial infarction. Treatment must cool the body to below 102 degrees as quickly as possible by ice water immersion since heat is lost from the skin very quickly by conduction to cold water. People with exertional heatstroke are quite sick, so ice water immersion should probably be done only when there are emergency medical personnel present to monitor the player. Obviously, most medical areas at local soccer competitions or tournaments are not equipped to treat heatstroke on site. Therefore, it is critical that athletes with heatstroke are transported to an emergency facility as quickly as possible. Cooling should begin before transport. Packing the entire body in towels that have been immersed in ice water is an effective first treatment. The more skin that is in contact with cold water, the more effectively heat will be lost. An older remedy was to place ice packs over the large vessels in the groin and axilla. However, this may result in a reflex constriction, so this older practice should probably be avoided. Spraying cool water on the skin and fanning air over the athlete may also be beneficial. Competitive venues must have methods in place to treat spectators as well, as they may not be acclimatized to the heat.

Prevention of Heat Illnesses

The risk of heat illnesses can be minimized by preparation prior to competition (acclimatization) and interventions (fluid ingestion), and there is some history of modifying the rules of a tournament to address heat illnesses.

Acclimatization is the gradual process of adapting to the local conditions. The process, while rapid, still can take 10–14 days of repeated exposure to the new, hotter climatic conditions. As the body adapts, sweating begins earlier, the sweat is more dilute because the body is conserving sodium, and there is a greater sweat rate. All of these changes increase the efficiency of heat loss and sodium conservation.

Fluid ingestion recommendations have been known for decades, and any team management personnel (coach, managers, trainers, doctors, parents) who restrict fluids during training may be courting a charge of negligence. The ACSM has very specific guidelines for fluid ingestion in managing heat problems.

Many people wrongly think that fluid ingestion during soccer is not possible due to the running clock. Remember that the ball is "in play" for only 60–70 minutes during a match (less in severe environmental conditions), so the wise use of injury stoppages and other times when the ball is out of play allows plenty of time for fluids. Plastic bottles can be placed in the goals, along the touch lines, or at the corners or carried out to the players during injury stoppages. During tournaments where postmatch drug screening is to be performed, each team can be given a designated color of plastic bottle. The laws of soccer are not an excuse for limiting fluid intake.

Another way to help keep players cool in the heat can be borrowed

In 1995 there were 500 youth teams from around the world at the U.S.A. Cup tournament in Blaine, Minnesota, in early July. Unfortunately, the heat and humidity were oppressive, with morning temperature and humidity both well into the 90s. In the first two days of competition there were fifteen players treated for heat illnesses. After two days of competition and all the treatments for heat, Dr. Bill Roberts, the head of the medical team, met with his group to discuss the heat problem. When the meeting broke, they took a recommendation to the tournament organizers to shorten each half by 5 minutes and to add the 5 minutes taken from the first half to halftime. Makes good sense, doesn't it? There would be a little shorter playing time and more time between halves to rehydrate without changing the overall schedule of the games. The organizers, however, decided not to make any changes. Dr. Roberts and his staff then elected to walk out of the tournament if the recommendations were not adopted. Faced with no medical coverage in dangerous weather conditions, the organizers relented and put the modifications in. The number of heat problems dropped dramatically over the rest of the weeklong tournament.

from American football. Most football sidelines will have a big water jug filled with ice water and towels. Put these towels over the head. With up to 40% of heat lost through the scalp, cold towels on the head are pretty effective. Plenty of leagues have free substitution, so there really are substantial opportunities to keep players cool. I have heard of people making their own mist tent or buying a liquid fertilizer dispenser from the hardware store and dedicating it to spraying water on players. I've even seen tournament organizers set up a mist tent like that seen at outdoor concerts. The attempt is to duplicate the effects of those misting fans seen on the sidelines of NFL games and others. Those fans are only effective if they are blowing hard enough; most of the homegrown methods may feel good but probably don't help the situation all that much.

There are other considerations regarding fluids and training:

- Thirst is a poor indicator of dehydration, so fluids must be encouraged even though the player does not feel thirsty.
- Dehydration limits performance. Players lose strength and endurance with as little as 2% weight loss due to dehydration (which can occur even *before* the player feels thirsty).

1 Drink 500 milliliters of cold water or fluid replacement beverage 90 minutes before competition.

2 Drink 150–200 milliliters every 15–20 minutes while competing. If the duration of competition is less than 1 hour, then water is probably the ideal fluid replacement beverage. If competition lasts more than 1 hour, then a carbohydrate/electrolyte solution (containing 4–8% carbohydrate) may be more beneficial.

3 After exercise, drink 1.5 liters of fluid replacement beverage per kilogram (or 1.5 pints per pound) of body weight lost during exercise.

- Humidity makes heat loss more difficult. Sweat evaporates down a gradient. The greater the gradient from the wet skin to the dry air (as in the desert), the faster the evaporation. The smaller the gradient (as in humid locations like the southeastern United States, Southeast Asia, the Indian subcontinent, and many others), the slower the heat loss and the greater the rise in body temperature, meaning more oppressive playing conditions.

- Extra salt is not necessary, as most athletes will naturally salt food according to taste. Salt tablets should never be offered or encouraged.

- Drinks with carbonation (like commercial sodas) for cooling should be avoided. The carbonation makes the athlete feel "full" sooner, meaning he or she will not drink the amount of fluid actually needed.

- Weighing before and after exercise is encouraged so that the desired amount of fluid can be consumed.

- Light clothing (in color and weight) is recommended. There are new moisture management materials available from most suppliers of athletic clothing that are very effective at assisting the body in evaporation and heat loss; they really are worth the extra expense.

- Overloading the player with water can lead to a dilution of body sodium, and this can be a serious problem. It is a mistake to think that a player can be prepared for the heat by having her drink *a lot* of water prior to play.

- All of these problems are magnified in children and the elderly. The symptoms of heat illness occur earlier in children and the elderly than in adults.

- All coaches, athletes, and parents must be educated about heat illness.

Competition in the Cold

Normal body temperature is much closer to the body's thermal "boiling point" than it is to its thermal "freezing point," so more emphasis is placed on heat problems. In many colder situations, behavioral strategies (e.g., clothing choices, shelter) are very effective at retaining heat. Most heat loss in the cold is by conductive and convective

For the 1969 national championship game, the Ohio State University football team showed up at the Rose Bowl wearing mesh jerseys. There had been some research done at the university showing just how much the uniform inhibited evaporation. Having played the end of the season in the Midwest, the players had lost some of the heat acclimatization they had gained earlier in the season. The temperature in Southern California was pretty hot that year, so the Buckeyes came prepared. Did it help? Who knows? They did win that game and the national championship.

Since then, clothing has been modified to aid in evaporation. The newest generation of clothing is termed "moisture management fabric" because the fluid evaporates from the new fiber faster than cotton. How? The fibers vary, but basically each fiber has channels along its length (cotton is cylindrical). This means that the newer fibers have more surface area exposed (some as high as 40% more surface area) to the air, allowing for faster evaporation of sweat. Coolmax and Dri-FIT are two of the most visible of these new materials. Read those labels!

mechanisms. Other environmental factors can influence heat loss in the cold, such as wind speed, solar radiation, and humidity. There is no one index of cold exposure like the WBGT, but the wind chill index (WCI) is widely accepted as a statement of cold stress. This index estimates the rate of cooling of a surface from the combined effects of temperature and wind. Wind chill tables are divided into zones that reflect the risk of freezing exposed tissues:

Little danger = above −30 degrees Celsius WCI
Moderate danger = between −30 degrees and −58 degrees
    Celsius WCI
Great danger = colder than −58 degrees Celsius WCI

While some might consider the concept of wind chill a very sound model, the formulas are constantly debated and revised. However, the WCI does help in making clothing decisions, as well as decisions about the advisability of holding an event.

The body responds to cold with a generalized vasoconstriction of the peripheral circulation to divert blood to the warmer core and an increase in the production of metabolic heat by shivering, a graded response to increasingly more severe cold. Exercise increases metabolic heat production far more than shivering. In the extremities there is an odd dilation of blood vessels due to oscillating skin temperature, which makes the fingers and toes most susceptible to cold injury. Plus, cold tends to contribute to a decline in manual dexterity. Cold-induced diuresis is a consequence of the redistribution of blood to the core. This means that, as in the heat, players need to be encouraged to drink fluids. Remember that during exercise, blood is diverted away from the kidneys, so exercise actually helps to minimize this diuresis. Body fat is an insulator and limits heat loss, so those with more body fat shiver less than their lean counterparts. In spite of the higher relative fat mass in women, they seem to be limited in their capacity to tolerate cold. As with the heat, the elderly and the very young are at greater risk for cold injury.

From a practical viewpoint, the soccer player performing in the cold may choose to wear a ski band to protect the ears and gloves to protect the hands and fingers. This is a common sight during winter competition. Players will probably also want to wear a layer or two underneath their club jersey. The layer closest to the skin should be a material that "wicks" sweat away from the skin to avoid excess skin cooling. Long training pants or running tights are not normally seen in soccer (although seen occasionally on the goalkeeper and referees). Players usually reject stretch hats as a nuisance to heading. Actually, the major concern at a match played in the cold is the spectators, as they may dress improperly (insufficient clothing or not dressing in bulk), fail to drink or drink the wrong beverages (e.g., alcohol, which will accelerate the diuresis), and are not exercising and may be relatively stationary for long periods in the cold.

Cold air affects heart rate response. When training at temperatures below 15 degrees Celsius (about 60 degrees Fahrenheit), the heart rate limits are said to be reduced by about 1 beat per minute per degree Celsius below 15. Thus, an activity that leads to a heart rate of 170 becomes 160 when training at 5 degrees Celsius.

Altitude

Any increase in altitude leads to a reduced partial pressure of oxygen: the percentage of air that is oxygen is the same; the molecules are just farther apart. Soccer can be contested at some severe altitudes like Mexico City (approximately 2,500 meters) or La Paz (approximately 3,600 meters). During a pool play match at the 1986 World Cup in

Mexico, the ball was in play for just over 45 minutes due to the altitude combined with the heat that day.

Altitude leads to a reduction in air resistance (or drag) and a reduction in oxygen transport by the blood, and it requires an acclimatization process. Endurance capacity falls with increased elevation beginning at about 1,200 meters. With increasing altitude, the driving pressure of oxygen into the blood is less, reducing the amount of oxygen carried by the blood, the subsequent unloading of oxygen due to a left shift of the oxyhemoglobin curve, and the ultimate delivery to the working muscle cells. In a game like soccer that has a large endurance component, the overall work output and intensity will be affected.

Acclimatization for competition to altitude requires planning. The medical team must realize first that exercise responses and time to acclimate are very individual. One player might have some difficulty with moderate altitude (approximately 1,500 meters), while another might have no problem. One player might adapt to an altitude quickly, and another might take twice as long. Fitness is no guarantee of protection against altitude sickness.

Chronic exposure to altitude stimulates multiple responses by the body to improve carriage, delivery, and use of oxygen, ultimately improving exercise performance. Ventilation, hemoglobin concentration, capillary density, mitochondrial number, and myoglobin (like hemoglobin, but in muscle) all adapt to improve oxygen use. Collectively, the adaptations improve submaximal performance. While the time course to adaptations can vary greatly among players, most adaptations will occur within 1–2 weeks, but some players might take much longer.

Because acclimatization improves performance at moderate altitude, the team should arrive at the site of competition 2–3 weeks early. This will maximize adaptation while minimizing the potential detraining that can occur with reduced training intensity. However, if the time for acclimatization is not available, some athletes find that arriving immediately prior to competition and then leaving right afterward seems to minimize the potential effects of the altitude. This procedure has not been scientifically tested. FIFA is holding a conference in October 2007 on high altitude matches, so watch for more on FIFA.com.

THE HIGHEST STADIUM IN THE WORLD

Pop quiz

What is the elevation of the highest stadium in the world?

Answer

Estadio Daniel A. Carrión in Cerro de Pasco, Peru, is at an incredible 4,380 meters, or 14,370 feet, where the temperature rarely is above 32 degrees Fahrenheit. There are only a handful of peaks in the Rockies above 14,000 feet; yet at this altitude in Peru there is a city of 70,000 people—with a professional soccer team.

Another consideration is training at altitude for performance at sea level. A team might want to hold a camp at altitude and then go directly to sea level for a match. The thought is that the altitude training would enhance endurance performance at sea level. A number of studies have been conducted on this concept, in an attempt to determine the best mix of training and altitude on subsequent sea-level performance. Currently, the best model appears to be the live high/train low theory. This concept combines the best of the adaptations from living at altitude (approximately 2,500 meters) with the ability to continue to train without reducing intensity at lower altitudes (approximately 1,250 meters). But practically, the logistics of travel each day make the model very challenging. Plus, some athletes may have sleep difficulties at moderate altitude. An alternative that has been tried is the so-called nitrogen house: an airtight house at sea level where the inside air is controlled to simulate altitude, and training is performed outside at sea level. Some people have tried a hypobaric bag (to simulate moderate altitude during sleep) or a hypoxic tent (same principle as the nitrogen house, just on a smaller scale). Research is continually under way on this concept to determine the optimal time exposure to altitude.

Air Pollution

With so many games and competitions occurring in major cities, the medical staff must address the issue of air pollution. Pollutants have both acute and chronic effects and come from mobile (e.g., automobiles) or stationary (e.g., industry) sources. Ozone, sulfur dioxide, carbon monoxide, lead, and fine particulate matter all can affect normal respiration and exercise performance.

Ozone. Ozone is produced by a photochemical reaction with the products of internal combustion engines. Symptoms of ozone exposure include cough, sore throat, substernal pain with a deep breath, and the feeling of a tight chest. Static pulmonary lung function values, as well as exercise performance, are decreased at values well below the daily ozone values seen in Mexico City, Los Angeles, and other cities with a high density of automobile traffic. There is an inverse, curvilinear relationship between ozone concentration and decrease in a standard test of lung function called the FEV$_1$ (forced expiratory volume in the first second; that is, the fraction of a maximal exhala-

POLLUTANTS IN MAJOR CITIES

Pollutant	Cities with High Levels
Ozone	Los Angeles, São Paulo, Mexico City, Houston
Sulfur dioxide	Pittsburgh, Seoul, Prague, Beijing, Mexico City
Particulate matter	Beijing, Shanghai, Bangkok, Mumbai
Nitrogen dioxide	Los Angeles, Athens, Mexico City, Moscow
Carbon monoxide	Mexico City

tion performed in 1 second). The asthmatic athlete has an aggravated (i.e., a smaller FEV_1) response, but exposure to ozone does not appear to aggravate athletes with exercise-induced asthma.

Carbon monoxide. Carbon monoxide is a product of internal combustion engines, as well as fires. Carbon monoxide binds reversibly with hemoglobin, reducing the oxygen content of the blood. Carbon monoxide combines with hemoglobin about 250 times faster than oxygen, making it more difficult to load the oxygen onto hemoglobin. Thus, the amount of oxygen carried, transported, and unloaded is reduced, and that will obviously reduce endurance performance. Cardiac patients are particularly at risk from carbon monoxide, not only because it lowers the oxygen content of the blood, but also because it can cause potentially fatal cardiac arrhythmias.

Sulfur dioxide. Sulfur dioxide is the result of the combustion of fossil fuels (e.g., at coal- and oil-fired power plants) and is also produced by refineries and pulp and paper mills. While sulfur dioxide will form acid aerosols and acid rain, exposure to typical levels will not impair respiration even in athletes working at very high intensities. But asthmatics likely will experience bronchoconstriction and wheezing even with very short exposures (i.e., 2–5 minutes). With the incidence of asthma in athletes being reported as high as 10%, the medical staff must be prepared for possible problems in their asthmatic athletes.

Nitrogen oxides. Nitrogen oxide is a primary exhaust emission, and nitrogen dioxide participates in the formation of ozone. The levels of each seen in the environment have little, if any, effect on respiration or exercise performance. However, exposure to nitrogen dioxide does increase respiratory illnesses in children.

Particulate matter. Particulate matters are small (approximately 15 micrometers in diameter) particles that come from many sources, such as dust, bacteria, pollen, and spores. Premature deaths have been reported during air pollution tragedies (e.g., the 1952 "London fog"). Patients with cardiovascular disease and chronic pulmonary disease are especially susceptible to particulate matter. Athletes training near heavily trafficked urban areas will likely inhale particulate matter during the mouth breathing needed to support high-intensity exercise.

Ozone and carbon monoxide can impair normal lung function and exercise performance. For the asthmatic, other pollutants can magnify the negative effects on exercise performance. In addition, patients with cardiac disease and chronic pulmonary conditions can have a higher mortality rate. The exposures to air pollutants that are a result of automobile traffic are the highest near the highways and dissipate with distance away from traffic.

CHAPTER 3

Injuries

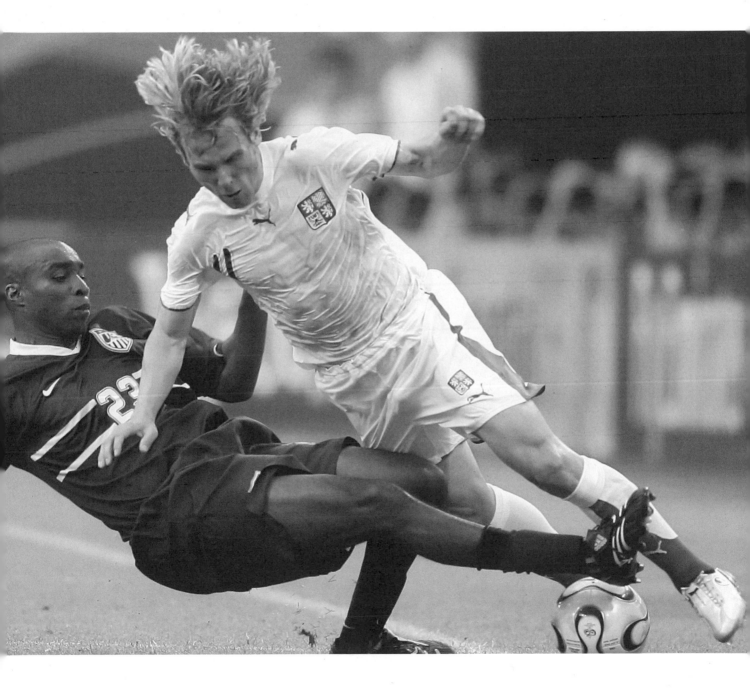

Sports injury research has taught us many things, some obvious, some not so obvious. We know that two-thirds of all injuries in soccer occur to the ankle, knee, head, leg, or foot. So, teams should be prepared to administer first aid for ankle and knee sprains, strained (pulled) muscles, contusions, lacerations, and concussions. Research has also shown us interesting things about the rate of injury in players with prior injuries. For example, about half the players with ankle sprains had a prior sprain, and many of those re-injuries happened in the same season. The risk of a sprain increases dramatically in players with a prior sprain. The question is not so much *if* you'll sprain that ankle again as much as it is *when* you will sprain that ankle again. Another important finding is that a major injury is often preceded by an incompletely rehabilitated minor injury—and that major injury doesn't necessarily happen to the same body part that had the minor injury.

Players and parents need to face facts: competitive sport is inherently risky, but that doesn't mean there is no way to protect players from injury. Here are some simple concepts of injury that might not be obvious to all. Most of these will be discussed in detail in this chapter.

- Poor flexibility and muscle tightness are often said to be a risk in muscle strains, tendon injuries, and muscle strain re-injuries. The knee extensors, hip flexors, and ankle dorsiflexors (which point your toe up) are known to be tight in soccer players. Therefore, don't neglect stretching these problem areas.
- An ankle sprain can happen while running on a poor surface, or it can happen by landing on someone's foot when coming down from a jump, like in basketball. Sprained ankles also happen during tackling, suggesting that technique may be an issue. Finally, ankle sprains can come from late tackles from the side when the tackler leaves his feet (a slide), which might indicate fair play issues. More critically, over half of those with an ankle sprain will re-injure that same ankle, and half of those do so within 2 months of the first injury. An ankle sprain is not just a nuisance injury like many players think. Follow the doctor's and therapist's orders about rehabilitation—they know what they are doing and know far more about it than players do. Returning too soon to play places the player at

When I talk about injuries, I like to use myself as an example to show that I know of what I speak. I started competing in sports in elementary school in the early 1960s playing Cub Scout softball. With such a long history of doing something that is inherently dangerous, I have had my share of injuries—I am a walking lab for a class on sports injuries. But nothing was career-ending. I'd RICE (rest, ice, compression, elevation), rehab, and return to play—to this day. So, as an introduction, I'd like to go through my injury history as best as I can remember. Given age and serendipity, this list is probably short; moreover, injury research shows most athletes remember, at best, about half of their injuries.

Cub Scout softball: While running back to the bench, I ran behind the backstop right into a kid swinging a bat. Outcome—broken incisor tooth (still evident).

High school track: Three injuries (that I can remember) and an illness: shin splints when we changed from a cinder to an asphalt track; bruised heel (I was a broad and triple jumper); pulled quadriceps muscle; mononucleosis (no doubt I had the bug in me that took hold after a hard workout that lowered my resistance).

Junior college track: Rebruised that heel a number of times.

Junior college soccer: Three injuries in one season: pulled right quadriceps (kept me from kicking with my right foot, so I learned to kick left-footed—in the end, a good thing); slight MCL (a knee ligament) sprain; and a slight LCL (the opposite knee ligament) sprain.

University track: I had one season of eligibility left so I tried to run track again. During winter training, I aggravated the LCL sprain from overexertion and had to quit track.

University soccer: Multiple sprained ankles (outdoors and indoors), strained groin muscles, one concussion.

Amateur soccer: Another concussion, strained groins, more sprained ankles, sprained MCL, two broken ribs (playing in a coed league against really weak players), separated shoulder (indoor league), partial retinal detachment (indoor league).

Basic fitness: Plantar fasciitis, twice—once that took me out of running for more than 2 years.

a clear risk for another, quite possibly more serious, injury to the ankle or elsewhere. Doctors and therapists recommend protecting an unstable ankle (e.g., taping, lace-up ankle supports) for *6 months to a year or more*. Do not to try to come back to play too soon. Follow rehabilitation guidelines completely to protect prior sprains or any injury. Players belong on the field, not on the sidelines.

· Risk factors for noncontact knee injuries include laxity, or loose ligaments, due to either prior injury or genetics; muscle imbal-

BASIC THOUGHTS ON INJURY

I never got injured playing soccer. I never played soccer. This is both simple and profound at the same time. Playing soccer, and all sports, has its risks. All those hours I did not spend at a sport that was not available where I grew up were spent playing football or baseball or driving a car. Going to the senior prom produced more dramatic injuries than playing soccer.

Many parents tell me that they prefer soccer to avoid the injury risk and rate of football. Actually, the injury rate is nearly identical. Parents ask at what age it is safe for their child to play football or soccer when, in fact, the risks of both increase dramatically with age from youth through high school. The risk also increases as players move up in intensity of play. There are fewer injuries to the recreational player than to the traveling player of the same age.

To paraphrase Forrest Gump, injuries do happen. Good medical attention can reduce the number of injuries, the severity of injuries, and the consequences of injury.

ance—one leg being stronger than the other, or the quads and hamstrings being imbalanced, which is usually due to weak hamstrings, not overly strong quadriceps (check out the Nordic curl exercise to improve hamstring strength later in this chapter); and problems of flexibility, since flexibility can reduce the risk of muscle strain injuries (though people with knee injuries generally have flexible hamstrings).

- Development of general motor skills is important in avoiding injury. Knee ligaments, the ACL (anterior cruciate ligament) in particular, seem to tear during landing from a jump, coming to a quick stop, or cutting. If any of these activities are done in an erect stance (straight knee and straight hip) and if there is some valgus (knock-kneed, X-legged, or "kissing knees," as the Europeans call it) at the knee, the strain on the ACL is drastically increased and can lead to a torn ligament. This is especially true in females. Players (women especially) are urged to play with a lower center of gravity and absorb the shock of landing by flexing the hips and knees; this means land softly and quietly and absorb the shock of impact at ground contact with the hips, knees, and ankles. For coaches, these are skills that should be taught when players are young. Puberty seems to be a reasonable age to start stressing these techniques. Before pu-

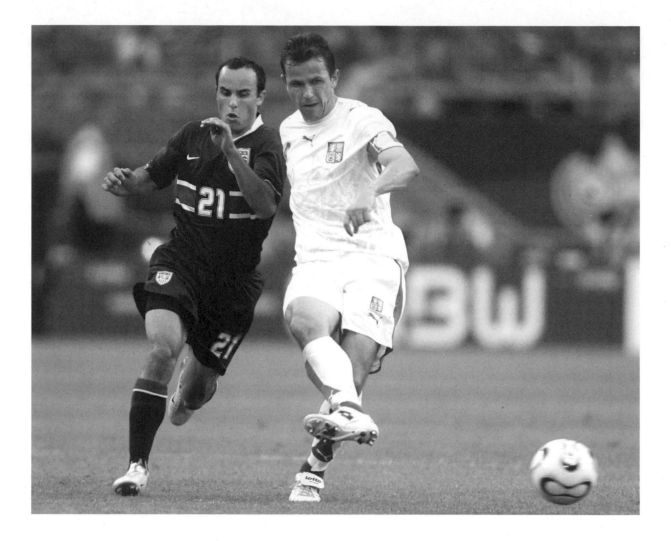

Tomas Galasek (right) and Landon Donovan, 2006 FIFA World Cup between
the United States and the Czech Republic. Most players focus flexibility on
their hamstrings and groin, but the hip shouldn't be neglected. Hip rotation is
needed for the simplest of skills. Preparing the foot to pass, as this Czech player
illustrates, requires significant outward rotation of his hip. Failure to do so
means an inaccurate pass. (Photograph by Tony Quinn; SoccerStock.com)

berty, boys and girls land, stop, and cut pretty much in the same way. As they get older, for some reason boys still absorb the shock of landing, while girls start to land stiff-legged. The typical female ACL patient these days is in middle school or high school.

- Low endurance clearly increases the risk of injury. Goals and injuries both tend to be concentrated late in the game, the time when player fitness becomes an issue. Injury surveys of both youth and professionals show that as much as 25% of all injuries occur in the last 10–15 minutes of a game. Many injuries from training happen during the preseason when players are not in condition. Ask any athletic trainer when players get hurt in training camp, and she will say during the last couple days of the week as players tire. You, the player, have a responsibility to arrive in shape—don't show up for camp to get in shape. Once in camp, the coach will improve everyone's fitness specifically for soccer, which will reduce fatigue later in the game.

- Soccer skill is also a factor in injury. Less-skilled players sustain more injuries. Skill work may seem dull, but we all know intuitively that the better-skilled players are injured less frequently. As an aside, my most painful injuries occurred when I was playing against opponents of lower ability: two broken ribs from an opponent who didn't realize he wasn't supposed to run into me after I passed the ball and a separated shoulder from an attempted tackle from behind that sent me cartwheeling right onto my shoulder. So in these cases, the cause of the injury was poor soccer ability, but the more experienced and skilled player, me, was the one who was hurt.

- Foul play has been implicated in injuries. Up to 50% of traumatic soccer injuries in elite men, and 25% in elite women, were due to foul play, sometimes to the "fouler," sometimes to the "foulee." Jumping into a player with both feet, usually from the side, leads to some pretty serious injuries. If a player has to leave her feet, she is out of position and desperate. Players should be taught not to leave their feet to tackle an opponent. Seeing these slides done by professionals doesn't make it right or a skill they should mimic.

- Middle school–age boys (approximately 11–14 years old) are a special case. During puberty, height increases faster than muscle growth. The tall, weak ("gangly") boy gets hurt more often than the shorter,

Soccer players generally have tighter muscles in their hip and thigh than most other athletes. Even with a reasonable flexibility program, the nature of soccer training may result in tighter muscle groups. There is good evidence that flexibility and strength training can lead to fewer injuries in those muscles most often injured. One key to proper muscle training is repeated measurement of strength and flexibility with simple field tests. An easy way to check flexibility is the simple toe-touch or the sit-and-reach test. These check how far one can reach toward or beyond the toes when either standing or sitting.

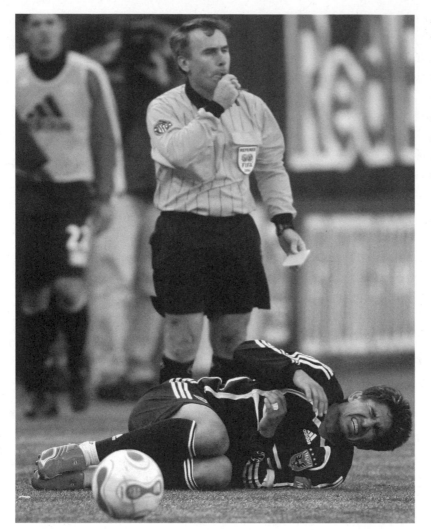

Jaime Moreno after a hard foul tackle from Amado Guevara, 2006 Major League Soccer playoffs between the D.C. United and the New York Red Bulls. A hard foul can lead to a serious injury as well as a private conversation with the referee. (Photograph by Tony Quinn; SoccerStock.com)

less mature boy or the taller, more mature boy. That "in-between" period is a problem because at this age, there is a wide range of maturity among players: some 14-year-olds are "going on 20," and some 13-year-olds still have the development of a 10-year-old.

• Shin guards are a required piece of equipment. All shin guards spread the impact across the guard, but don't think a shin guard is there to prevent fractures. When the kicking equivalent of a sledge-hammer comes in contact with the leg, the shin pad will probably not prevent a fracture. Shin guards that spread out the impact the best are made of air/foam-filled pads; these also happen to be the largest pads on the market. Most players want the bare minimum to pass the referee's inspection. It should be obvious that the larger the shin guard, the more protection it affords. I recall watching a professional team in training. When it was time to scrimmage, the bulk of the players put on children's shin pads because they are small and light. There is a big problem with using small shin guards, however: they don't protect the part of the leg that takes the brunt of the collisions. Most contusion injuries happen to the bottom third of the leg—the unprotected area. Look at the players during any professional or national team game on TV, or at photos on the websites of FIFA, U.S. Soccer, or your favorite team. Small shin pads are worn on the upper half of the leg. Law IV only states that a player must wear shin guards, with no qualifying statements on size. (Could a reinterpretation of Law IV be coming? You never know.) Leg contusions can be minimized by wearing age-appropriate shin guards. Beginning in 2007, the governing body of U.S. high school sports requires age-appropriate shin guards.

- Head injuries occur during head-elbow, head-head, or head-ground contact, mostly near the midline (when competing for goal kicks, punts, clears, etc.) and sometimes in the penalty area (when competing for crosses). Especially dangerous are head flicks where a player flicks the ball off the head, usually backwards. If the player who wants to head the ball does not separate from the defender, there is danger to both players—the defender behind who jumps for the head can get hit on the chin or on the nose by the first player or the player who heads the ball can get hit in the back of the head. For example, a player throws into a teammate's head who must head (flick) the ball over her own head. The defender jumps to head the ball. A whiplash-type injury is being set up here. Jumping slightly, the player receiving the throw impacts the ball and the opponent's face/nose/chin, leading to possible fractures plus a concussion from the impact and whiplash. This can be prevented by a few coaching points. Teach the player receiving the ball either to take a step back to control the ball with the chest/thigh/foot (the ref won't make a call for this) or head it back to the thrower or other visible teammate. Or, teach the thrower to throw the ball so that it can be controlled easily (to the feet, thigh, or chest instead of the head). Throwing the ball (legally) to a teammate's feet takes some practice—it isn't as easy as it sounds. This option protects

Shin guards do not have the ability to prevent most of the fractures seen in the legs of soccer players. However, they can and do stop many of the injuries and much of the time lost from practice and games due to contusions or bruising. They are just as valuable in practice as in games. The clever coach knows to insist on shin guards in all practice situations where an opponent is involved. No need to wear shin guards while stretching or doing individual ball skills training.

both players and is better tactically. In the overwhelming number of cases, the player has no idea where that flick is going anyway, so it is just a wasted pass. Despite its simplicity, the throw-in is a skill and a tactic that needs practice.

• A fractured wrist in young goalkeepers is a preventable injury. This happens when an adult shoots an adult (size 5) ball at young goalkeepers. Always use the age-appropriate ball, and only have players the same age take real shots on goal. This is just common sense. Coaches may think they are helping their young keeper, but they are really increasing the risk of a wrist, hand, or finger injury.

• Another completely preventable (and gruesome) finger injury is called a "degloving" injury. Think about that phrase. Before games, nets need to be put on the goals, and many goals have hooks in the crossbar for the nets. This injury happens when someone jumps to put the net over a hook in the bar and catches a ring on the hook. Gravity then takes over. See how it gets its name now? Can you picture the ugly result? Never jump. Always stand on a ladder or other suitable support.

• Finally, goalpost injuries to children have led to catastrophic neck injuries and some deaths. These happen when unsupervised children climb on portable goals, and the goal tips over on a child. *Portable goals should always be secured to the ground*, and children should *never* be allowed to play on goals. All fatalities of this sort have occurred outside of games when children were unsupervised. FIFA clearly states that no goal should ever be left unsecured.

Many soccer injuries, especially re-injuries, are preventable. Physical preparation prior to play is as important as decisions made during play. The main objective of any physical training program is to improve physical function so that the player can perform at a higher level than before *and* be protected against injury.

YOUTH INJURIES

In the late 1990s, while working at Duke Sports Medicine, we undertook a 3-year survey of Classic League soccer players in North Carolina. The Classic League is the highest level of traveling play in the state. Nike was the driving force behind this substantial project. Over

HEADING VERSUS HEAD INJURY

Head injury, including concussions, is the hot topic among soccer governing bodies from the local recreational leagues all the way to FIFA. There have been allegations that the impacts of "heading" have cumulative effects and lead to cognitive dysfunction — kind of like the sum of all those jabs a boxer absorbs without ever being knocked out. A number of research studies on soccer players do not show a long-term effect on mental functioning even at very high level players (collegiate and professional). Most people in sports medicine do not believe that purposeful heading is an issue in the cognitive dysfunction seen in a small number of players.

However, there is more concern now about concussions, which may or may not occur in the act of heading. Concussions most often involve head-to-head, -elbow, or -ground contact, not purposeful head-to-ball contact (accidental head-to-ball contact can lead to a concussion). Medical professionals have two pretty big problems when it comes to a head injury: recognizing the injury (remember, loss of consciousness is not a requirement for a concussion) and knowing when to allow a player to return to sports. Current research to determine when a player's mental function returns to normal after a concussion should help doctors make better-informed decisions on the return to play. A sound decision in this matter is critical to reduce the risk of re-injury or of making the current injury worse.

PROTECTING THE KEEPER

Soccer goalkeepers usually practice as long as the field players and will field an indeterminate number of shots. Stopping a shot without injury requires highly developed motor skills. Most youngsters or unskilled players have little idea about the energy in a driven shot. Hand and wrist injuries are common even in skilled keepers; a coach or parent must control shooting situations, especially when an overzealous attacker is shooting on an occasional goalie.

UNSECURED GOALS

Unfortunately, an analysis of serious injuries and deaths in soccer shows that far too many children are hurt by unsecured goals. Team physicians do not see or talk about these injuries too often, so parents, coaches, and team and league administrators must take the lead.

3 years we ended up working on a database of over 20,000 players statewide.

We were interested in the type, frequency, and mechanism of injuries among these players. Most parents, coaches, and players don't read the journals where this kind of information is found, so here is a bulleted summary of some of our findings:

• 94% of the injuries happened during competition. This may be because there were so few practices each week (typically two)

This is for those parents who have some soccer-playing experience. If you have a playing history, you probably also have an injury history. Ever wonder if you will be paying for your passion in the years to come? The short answer is probably, somewhere.

Concussions: The big question, largely unanswered to this point, is whether purposeful heading has any effect on cognitive function. Yes, there is good evidence that a small fraction of soccer players have some cognitive deficits. No, there is no convincing evidence that purposeful heading is at the root of such deficits. There are lots of reasons why, beyond just purposeful heading, a player might have some problems with concentration and short-term memory. The main culprit is concussions. Having had one concussion might not be an issue. Multiple concussions are of greater concern: in particular, sustaining multiple injuries with a short time between injuries is most likely the reason for lingering cognitive problems. You know that neurologists everywhere want to see how football players with multiple concussions like Troy Aikman and Steve Young will be doing in the coming years.

Neck arthritis: If purposeful heading has some lingering effects, people are probably looking for them a little too far north, so to speak. Retired players in their forties and fifties have arthritis in their neck at around five times the rate of the public. It appears that compression on the neck has led to bone spurs, arthritis, and reduced range of motion. Neck arthritis is seen in around 15% of retired soccer players, so this, as most things, doesn't happen to everyone.

Hip arthritis: While hip injuries are pretty rare in soccer players, hip arthritis also affects around 15% of retired players, which is a far greater rate than experienced by the general public. I have teammates younger than I who have had total hip replacements. If you see a couple of career coaches in their fifties talking together at some meeting, they might just as well be discussing their hip surgery as tactics. The mechanism for such a high rate is unknown.

Knee arthritis: Again, I know former teammates now with artificial knees. The overall incidence of knee arthritis in retired soccer players has not been reported. One of the main reasons for knee arthritis is a prior knee injury, particularly an injury to the meniscus or the ACL. Recent reports have shown that an injury to a meniscus means an earlier onset of osteoarthritis. The same goes for an ACL tear; whether or not you have surgery, the chances are very good that within 15 years, you will have signs or symptoms of arthritis.

Ankle instability: The ankle is the most injured joint in soccer players. Ankle instability from multiple sprains and contusions means that with time, ankle range of motion will decline, and arthritis will creep in.

I am not trying to throw any fear into you parents with a playing history. As I have said, sports are inherently dangerous, and it's the injuries, not the sport, that lead to future problems. The problems don't happen to all retired players. Some played for years and were never injured, so they are unlikely to have any lingering problems. No study has ever shown that exercise alone is a risk of future arthritis. Some players played for years, had some injuries, and still didn't have any problems. Finally, there is no evidence that any of these lingering issues has any effect on the normal activities of daily living. Not every player will develop problems—besides, I am guessing that most people in middle age don't regret a second of their playing careers.

or because of the competitive nature of the games in the Classic League.

- 63% of all injuries were to the leg, 15% to the head and neck, 11.5% to the trunk, and 10% to the arm. Not all the head injuries were concussions. Many were lacerations and other minor injuries.
- Almost 90% of the time, the injured player was held out of play, but medical care was sought for fewer than half the injuries. The decision to leave the field was usually made by the player.
- Contact was involved in nearly 70% of all injuries. The rest had no player-to-player contact.
- Most injuries were minor, as 60% of all players missed less than 1 week out of play or practice. One week is usually the cutoff between minor and more serious injuries.
- Most people think flexibility is important in preventing injury. We asked the injured players how far they could reach when asked to touch their toes, and 10% of the boys could reach only to their shins yet over half the girls could place either their knuckles or palms on the floor. Fewer than 30% of the boys could reach that far.
- Three-quarters of the injured girls did regular flexibility training. Fewer than half the boys did regular flexibility training.
- The overwhelming majority (94%) of players wore molded sole shoes at the time of injury (many of the fields in North Carolina are really too hard for screw-in studs or so-called soft ground shoes).
- One in 5 injured players wore an in-shoe insert or orthotic. (It is getting to the point where sports shoes are a shell in which you insert your own custom orthotic—there is no way sport shoe makers can make a shoe that fits all foot types.)
- One in 20 players wore a mouth guard.
- Plastic or osi shin pads were worn by 75% of the players.
- A foul was called in about 20–25% of the injuries.
- In the cases where a foul was not called, a quarter of the injured players thought a foul should have been called.
- Defenders (including the goalkeeper) sustained nearly half the total number of injuries. Midfielders and forwards equally split the remaining injuries. These numbers were the same for both boys and girls.

from the Team Doc

A COUPLE OF OBSERVATIONS ABOUT ARTHRITIS

Even though retired professional players have a higher incidence of arthritis, it is usually not severe or disabling. It is probably true that knee injuries especially accelerate the "normal" arthritis process seen with aging. Remember, the running, jumping, and training associated with sports like soccer do not seem to produce the arthritic changes—those seem to come from a discrete injury.

- The contusion rate was about the same for boys and girls.
- Ice was the most common first aid, but 20% said they did not seek any treatment.
- Contusions are usually minor injuries, as 54% with these injuries missed no games or practice and 80% missed 1 week or less.
- Contusions were about equally split between the halves of play. Other injuries happen as players get tired, but not contusions.
- Most injuries occurred on the ball (82%); the player usually fell (63%); and few could stay on and continue (20%). They came off and were treated with ice.

THE MOST DANGEROUS PART OF THE GAME

I always say that players and coaches need to know more about their game, more than just skills, certainly more than just tactics. You need to know when to run, when to stop, when to play fast, when to play slow (University of North Carolina men's coach Elmar Bolowich has told me a major weakness of American players is they don't know how and when to play slow), when to tackle, when to back up, when to shoot, and when to pass. Players need options, and they need to know when to use those options so they aren't predictable robots who only know Route 1 soccer. The ability to execute options is what makes soccer so attractive and fun.

It makes sense that if a player or coach knows how an injury happens, then maybe the player can avoid that injury when such a situation occurs. So here is my question: What is the most dangerous part of the game? Heading? Running? Tripping? The professional foul?

A number of studies about how injuries occur have been conducted. For example, knee injuries can result either from direct contact or from an awkward misstep while cutting or landing. Head injuries often happen while competing for a head ball. They usually involve elbow-head contact for men and head-head contact for women. Ankle injuries can be the result of stepping on another player's foot or from unequal forces during a tackle. Shin injuries often occur in close quarters while tackling. Foot injuries happen when a player reaches for the ball during a tackle, and the opponent steps on that foot. A broken tibia or fibula can result from a hard kick to the shin during tackling.

I hope you see the pattern. The most dangerous activity in soccer is tackling. More injuries occur during tackling than during any other activity. Any number of reasons can be offered. For example, with players with mismatched skills, the better player could be cut down by the lesser player. Some of my worst injuries were from playing recreational ball with unskilled, inexperienced players.

Some people think tackling is something innate in a player; you either are or are not a good tackler. The coach who thinks this is true probably spends little time teaching and practicing the skill of tackling—a very big mistake.

When I took the U.S. Soccer coaching school (back when it was new), team defense and defensive priorities in man marking were an important part of the course. While these concepts have evolved with time, you will get the idea. As a team, the priority is to protect penetration of a player, ball, or both. As a defender, my hierarchy of defense was:

1 Cover the player in my area so well that his teammates won't think about passing the ball to that player.
2 If a pass is made, step up and intercept the pass.
3 If the pass can't be intercepted, pressure the player so he can't turn around—forcing a back pass.
4 If the player does turn, keep the player and the ball in front of you. Jockey and shepherd the player to a less dangerous part of the field or to a position in which the player is less of a threat.
5 Finally, go for the tackle.

Tackling was the last option. Of all the ways a team can obtain possession of the ball, tackling is about fourth or fifth on the list. Some might say, "OK, then why teach tackling? It's a low priority for getting the ball." Yet tackling is where the bulk of injuries occur. The top three locations for injuries in soccer are the ankle, knee, and shin. Doesn't tackling look like a problem now? Current FIFA research shows that there is a higher risk of injury during two-footed tackles, especially from the side. At the level of play in the FIFA studies, a tackle from behind was a low risk for injury mostly because of the severe penalty (ejection) for bringing down a player from behind—a clear example of how rule interpretation and enforcement have legislated out a particular style of tackle. I wouldn't be surprised if in the future tackles in which a player leaves his feet (especially with spikes up) suffer a

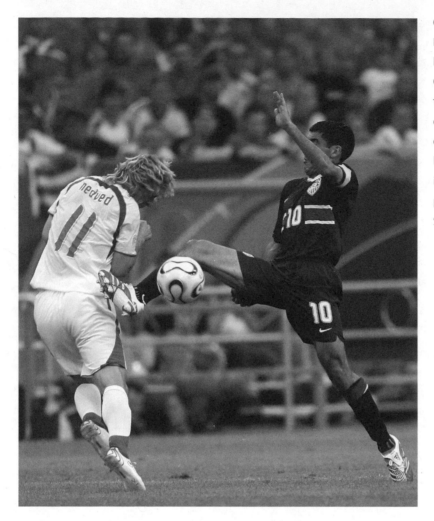

Claudio Reyna (right) and Pavel Nedved, 2006 FIFA World Cup between the United States and the Czech Republic. A studs-up challenge from the side is one of the most dangerous tackles in soccer. Not only can it cause serious injuries, but opponents remember these incidents and sometimes attempt payback. (Photograph by Tony Quinn; SoccerStock.com)

similar sanction. Refs at the 2006 World Cup were given the authority to eject such offenders.

A clash of heads also carries a high risk of injuries. FIFA research shows that most head injuries occur in the midfield, not in front of the goal. Midfield head injuries happen when two players, coming from opposite directions, both jump for the ball into each other, and heads collide, or an elbow or hand strikes a temple, subjecting one or both heads to a rotational, twisting motion that is particularly dangerous. Injury is not all that frequent when two players both jump straight up for a ball. If an injury does occur, it is usually linear and not as dangerous as a rotational injury. In the penalty area, players just don't get the same run-up on the ball. Watch for these situations during games,

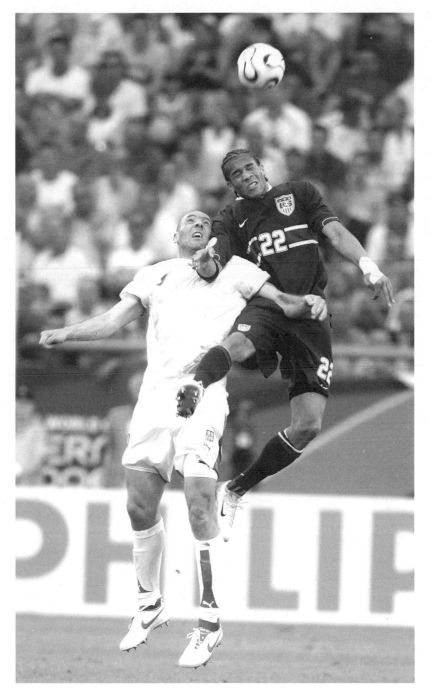

Oguchi Onyewu (right) and Jan Koller, 2006 FIFA World Cup between the United States and the Czech Republic. An elbow-to-head impact can lead to a very dangerous rotational head injury and concussion. Such a collision usually happens in the open field as two players approach from different directions. If the referee feels the use of the elbow was intentional, a red card can be shown. (Photograph by Tony Quinn; SoccerStock.com)

and you can see it coming. It's safer to stay on the ground or jump straight up. Besides, the first touch on an air ball isn't the important touch. Coaches constantly stress that the second touch on an air ball is the important touch.

Whenever jumping into a player is involved, the risk of injury increases. When players stay on their feet while tackling, fewer injuries result. The most important thing that a player can learn is to stay on her feet when she tackles. If a player leaves her feet to tackle, she is probably out of position and a bit desperate. When players leave their feet to tackle, bad things can happen to both players.

While tackling is not something any one player performs all that frequently during a game, it is a skill to be practiced, practiced, practiced. When players practice tackling, they become more comfortable on the ball and are prepared to attempt a tackle with confidence, so they can concentrate on the ball and not get distracted. Practice activities in small-sided games give more opportunity for tackling practice.

MUSCLE INJURY: THE "PULLED MUSCLE" AND DELAYED MUSCLE SORENESS

Doctors, trainers, and therapists see common muscle injuries, including contusions, lacerations, strains, and complete tears. These injuries lead to significant pain and disability, with time lost from sports and other activities. Muscle strains, or what most athletes call a "pulled muscle," can account for nearly 30% of the injuries seen in a typical sports medicine practice.

There are a number of noncontact injuries that can affect muscle function. Probably the most common is called delayed onset muscle soreness (DOMS). During unaccustomed exercise, eccentric loading leads to microscopic damage to the cells. The damage is felt as local pain (DOMS), weakness, and reduced range of motion. Pain usually peaks in the 1–2 days following exercise. Weakness and limited range of motion can last for over a week.

A fascinating part of DOMS is how fast the muscles adapt. Do the same exercise again, and the perceived soreness is less, and there is less tissue damage. Do the same exercise again, and the soreness is even less.

In a muscle strain injury, there is damage to the area where the muscle and tendon join together. The pain can be almost anywhere along the length of the muscle, but the damage still is at the muscle-tendon junction (this is an anatomy issue—tendons reach way up into muscles, not what you might draw if asked to illustrate the tendon-muscle-tendon). Perform an activity that uses the damaged muscle, and there is local pain and general weakness of the muscle, designed to prevent further damage. Improper rest and poor rehabilitation of a minor injury like a muscle strain frequently precedes a more serious and disabling injury.

Mechanism of Muscle Injury

A muscle strain is usually predictable. Specific muscles under certain circumstances will strain. What happens is somewhat complicated. Two things must occur. First, obviously the muscle must be contracting, but second, there must be some lengthening of the muscle while it is trying to shorten. The weak point in the system is where two distinctly different tissues unite—at the junction of the muscle and the tendon. Microscopic tears are seen across the muscle. When there is now damage between the muscle and tendon, the muscle can't develop tension the way it is supposed to. When you try to contract the muscle, you feel pain. Depending on the severity of the tear, bleeding can be visible as a bruise under the skin but still within the fascia surrounding the compartment. Fatigue is a factor in strain injury, as it is in so many injuries. Many strains happen late in the game. Obviously, the larger the injury, the poorer the prognosis.

A strained muscle usually occurs during sprinting or when stretching to reach a ball. The design of certain muscles puts them at risk for a strain injury. Typically, the muscles most vulnerable in the soccer player are the hamstrings (mostly the biceps femoris—the one on the outside of the back of the thigh), the rectus femoris (the middle muscle of the thigh), and a certain groin muscle (adductor longus). Other muscles can sustain a strain injury, but in running sports, these are the main muscles at risk. Injury to the hamstrings can occur during sprinting, to the rectus during sprinting and kicking (for example, dragging your toes into the ground when shooting), and to the groin when stretching to the side during a tackle.

from the Team Doc

TACKLING AND INJURY

From the standpoint of the team physician near the bench, it is amazing how the perception of tackling varies with age and skill level. Youth players (and mostly their vocal parents) think every tackle is a deliberate rule violation and should be punished. In their teen years, the same players want to be sure to inflict as many hard tackles on the opponents as the opponents inflict on them ("You *tackled* me? I got your number!"). The most skillful players look to avoid a tackle and gain an advantage by playing the ball past a defender.

In treating injuries due to tackling, it is clear that the attacker and defender are at similar risks. I have seen more tibia fractures in the defensive player than in the player being tackled.

Muscle develops tension in two ways.

Concentric contraction: This is what most people think of when they think of how a muscle works. The muscle builds up tension and overcomes the resistance on the limb by shortening, and the joint moves.

Eccentric contraction: By this method the muscle develops tension while lengthening. When you do a forearm curl, you contract the biceps (and two other muscles, called the brachialis and brachioradialis). When you lower the bar, you do not contract the triceps; you allow the biceps and brachialis to slowly lengthen, still developing tension. Eccentric contractions are critical in controlling limb movements during landing from a jump and changing directions while running.

There is an interesting difference between the two types of contractions. Just for descriptive purposes, let's say it takes 100 cells (fibers) to lift 100 pounds concentrically. To lower the weight, it might take only 10 fibers to lower the 100 pounds (and gravity isn't as big a factor as you might think). What this means is that during a concentric contraction, the tension per fiber is 1 pound (100 pounds/100 fibers), while during the eccentric contraction the tension per fiber is 10 pounds (100 pounds/10 fibers). During eccentric contractions, then, each fiber that is working is working harder than during a concentric contraction.

Rehabilitation and Repair

A strained muscle is what some call a self-limiting injury, meaning you just ride out the pain and, eventually, the muscle will heal. Typically, there is progressive loss of strength over the next day or two following the injury, then strength begins to return gradually. An ice compression bandage should be applied immediately after the injury as this hastens recovery. More severe injuries might require the use of crutches, but most players will alter their gait to protect the painful muscle. Just watch how a person with a pulled groin walks or negotiates stairs. As the pain decreases, some mild range of motion exercises and stretching will be suggested. Once nearly full range of motion has returned (there is some scarring in the muscle), mobility exercises are begun. With pain-free movement, jogging and running can be added. A player needs to have full range of movement, returned strength, and full function to return to play. Pain medications help some people, but no pill helps heal the tissue any faster than nature. Most people return to practice in 1–2 weeks, unless the injury is really severe. Surgery is needed if the muscle tears completely away from the bone (if you follow Reds baseball, this is what happened to Ken Griffey Jr. in 2004).

The question went something like this: "My 12-year-old son plays club soccer and has pain below his kneecap and above his shin when he plays soccer or goes up and down stairs. Someone used the term 'Osgood-Schlatter's disease.' What is this disease? Is this what he has?"

This parent's first mistake was to ask this question of a non-M.D. like myself. Always consult a physician. But Osgood-Schlatter's disease is the most common cause of knee pain in adolescents, particularly in boys. It can happen in one or both knees. The pain is found on that bump just south of the kneecap. This is where the tendon of the quadriceps (thigh) muscle inserts into the tibia at the tibial tubercle (that "bump"). This is also the area of the tibial growth plate, which is where the bone increases in length. When a child starts his growth spurt in adolescence and plays sports requiring running and jumping, the repetitive high-force demands by the quadriceps can pull on the bony insertion on the tibia. This may lead to a partial pulling away of the tendon from the bone (called an avulsion). If the syndrome progresses, a partial gap can form that can be filled with fibrous tissue instead of bone, and this can also be painful. The body attempts to repair the damage by reworking the tissue back into bone, which can lead to a very prominent tibial tubercle—a more pronounced knot.

What usually brings a child to the doctor is swelling and tenderness at the tibial tubercle. The tubercle may be enlarged, and pain can be induced with direct pressure or strong quadriceps contractions, like in jumping. Using stairs can also be painful. X-rays may or may not be ordered.

The treatment for Osgood-Schlatter's disease is what is called symptomatic: treat the symptoms. When pain develops, the athletic trainer's axiom of RICE is the treatment of choice: *Rest* (from painful activity), *Ice* (3 x 20 minutes a day), *Compression* (with a knee sleeve or "ace" bandage), and *Elevation* (elevate the leg). If the pain continues, the doctor may suggest a brace that reduces tension on the tendon.

from the Team Doc
OSGOOD-SCHLATTER'S DISEASE

This condition is usually considered to be self-limiting. The young athlete can continue to play, even with some discomfort, without bringing on a poor outcome. It is possible that activity needs to be limited to control the symptoms. Often, the parents have more symptoms than the child, and a thorough explanation of the condition may be enough to relieve anxiety of the parent and child.

Aspirin or ibuprofen may be effective at reducing pain and swelling. Crutches will take the load off the leg. Several weeks or months may be needed for pain to cease. In other words, a young player could be symptomatic for an entire season. The doctor might prescribe some exercises, like straight leg raises, quadriceps contractions, and leg curls, to strengthen these leg muscles. Ice should be used after exercise to minimize pain and swelling. Those Nordic curls (the hamstring strengthening exercise) in the F-MARC 11 probably should be avoided.

In most children, Osgood-Schlatter's will go away with rest and time. Ignoring the pain or playing through the pain puts the player at risk of making the condition worse, leading to much longer time out of sports. As the growth rate slows, the tendon becomes stronger. This condition rarely persists beyond the growth stage.

HEAD INJURIES

Soccer is unique because of the purposeful use of the unprotected head to control and advance the ball. This places the head in a vulnerable position for numerous types of injuries. The head and neck make up about 15% of the surface area of the body and sustain a similar proportion of the total injuries seen in soccer. Head injuries are almost exclusively due to acute trauma from collisions with other players, the ground, the ball, or the goal. When the topic of head injuries comes up, I hate it when the press says that "soccer players can kick a ball 60–70 miles per hour." They can—but when they do, most players in the path of the ball will duck. Watch games at any level: when the ball is coming fast, players duck.

The most common serious head injury is a concussion, sometimes called a mild traumatic brain injury (MTBI). A concussion is simply any alteration of normal brain function, but a full definition is quite involved. The general public seems to think that one needs to be unconscious to have sustained a concussion, and this just isn't true. If you see a player collide heads with another player, and one or both are wandering around seemingly unaware of what is going on around them, they probably have had concussions and need to be removed from the game. I have talked with colleagues on other continents who say they don't have a concussion problem. Of course they do. What they have also is a concussion recognition problem. In the 2004 Copa America final between Brazil and Argentina, a Brazilian defender was obviously knocked unconscious when he and an Argentine striker collided heads. The Brazilian was out cold from the time of contact all the way to the ground and for some time afterward—and he was left in the game only to be removed from the game maybe 5–10 minutes later and then transported out of the stadium by ambulance. He is fine. However, this player should never have been allowed back in the game.

Minor or Rare Head Injuries

Accidental contact to the head can lead to a number of injuries. The most common minor injury is the same as to the legs—a contusion/abrasion injury. The player might not be paying attention to the game and get a ball to the face. Or an errant ball might hit her before she can get out of the way. Upon contact, there is the chance the skin can be broken, leading to a laceration. As with any sport, open bleeding must be addressed immediately, and the player can't return to play until the bleeding is controlled, and any exposed blood on the player or uniform is removed. One of the most common lacerations seen in soccer is to the mouth, especially to teenagers who have orthodontic braces and no mouth guard. While the Laws of the Game don't require mouth protection, at the very least, players with braces should wear some form of mouth protection. See a dentist for suggestions. In addition, a common and dangerous head injury occurs during a flick-on header, when the player flicking the ball ends up hitting the chin of the defender, causing a whiplash injury. There are many who suggest wearing mouth protection as a preventive measure against this kind of injury because much of the force from the heading player is absorbed by the mouth guard. Scientific data to support the value of a mouth guard in preventing a concussion, however, is lacking. One can get guards at a sports store that offer some protection, but a dentist is far wiser in selecting and fitting a device than is a store sales associate.

Lacerations to the scalp get everyone's attention because of the amount of bleeding, due to the dense blood supply to the scalp. Although in many cases they appear to be worse than they really are, all scalp injuries obviously need immediate attention and possible follow-up in an emergency room.

I see this frequently, especially in the women's game. An air ball comes to a player and, not knowing what to do with the ball, she flicks the ball off the top of her head (with or without a small jump), deflecting the ball over the back of her head. I know you have seen this.

This move brings dangers to both the player and the defender. The defender, while trying to head the ball, can get hit in the face or chin by the player in front, causing a whiplash injury. I have even seen fractured noses or cheeks. Meanwhile, the attacker can get hit in the back of the head by the defender.

Coaching the Situation

I put on my coaching hat for these tips:

- When players pass the ball in the air, aim for the space in front of the receiver so she can control the ball with the feet. If she chooses to try and head the ball, she must separate from the defender by running to meet the ball with the head instead of standing and waiting for the ball.

- On a throw-in, players should throw the ball to feet as opposed to the head. This takes some practice. Or throw to the chest or thigh. The receiver should attempt to move to a place with open ground for the thrower to aim for. If the ball does come to the head, the receiver should push the defender back a little and head the ball back to the thrower, or receive the ball with the feet, thigh, or chest.

On the Value of a Flick-On Header

My opinion is that most flick-on headers are a wasted pass. It happens because the player has no clue on what her options are. The flick-on headers that "work" are those where the heading player runs to the ball, separating herself from anyone behind. For example, on a corner driven to the near post, the player moves quickly to the ball and lets the ball skip off her head to the far post. She doesn't stand and wait for the ball.

Eye injuries are very scary. What usually happens is a hard kick sends the ball into the face of a player who is unable to avoid contact (I am speaking from experience on this one). The eye is protected pretty well by the bony cave of six bones that it sits within, and the soccer ball, unlike, say, a racquetball, is too big to make direct contact with the eye. However, when the ball strikes the face, the impact can lead to fracture of any of the bones or injury to the soft tissues of the eye. When eye injuries happen, there is little discussion: the player is removed and likely taken to a hospital—and an eye injury is one of a few conditions that moves the patient to the front of the line at the emergency room.

In my case, a defender I was pressuring from behind pivoted to clear the ball instead of passing back to the keeper as I expected, and the ball struck me square on the face. The force popped a small hole in my retina. The injury happened on a Wednesday night, the emergency room doctor got me an appointment with an ophthalmologist for Thursday, and I had surgery on Friday. There was no damage to my contact lens, and a small bruise on my eyelid was the only visible sign of injury. I have learned to live with a small, out of the way, blind spot.

Concussion

The jokes can be heard along the sidelines or in the stands most anywhere in the country. When a player heads a ball, someone is bound to say, "Well, there goes ten points on his SAT," or "Scratch Harvard off the list." These seemingly harmless jokes belie a real concern of soccer parents: heading and head injuries in soccer.

I once watched Germany score six of eight goals against Saudi Arabia with headers. In 2003 the leading scorer in Algeria died following complications when he landed head first after losing his balance in the air while competing for a head ball. Such examples raise a number of questions: Are there dangers from purposeful ball-to-head contact? Are there dangers from accidental ball-to-head contact? How dangerous is it for the head when contacting a hard surface like another player's head, foot, or elbow? These questions have led to the consideration of head protection in soccer.

Mechanism of injury. Purposeful heading does not appear to be the real issue in discussions of mild traumatic brain injury. I can't recall any player being concussed from *purposeful* heading of a ball, but it may have happened when a player tried to head, rather than avoid, an extremely hard shot. A concussion from purposeful heading prior to the introduction of the water-resistant ball (in the early to mid-1970s) was possible because the old leather ball could gain up to 20% or more in water weight when the game was played in the rain. (Most modern balls absorb little water, but simply using a new ball is no guarantee against injury. If a ball gets noticeably heavier when wet, replace it before the next session.) Practically all concussions are caused by head contact with some other hard object, such as another head, an elbow, a foot, knee, goalpost, or the ground. In women's soc-

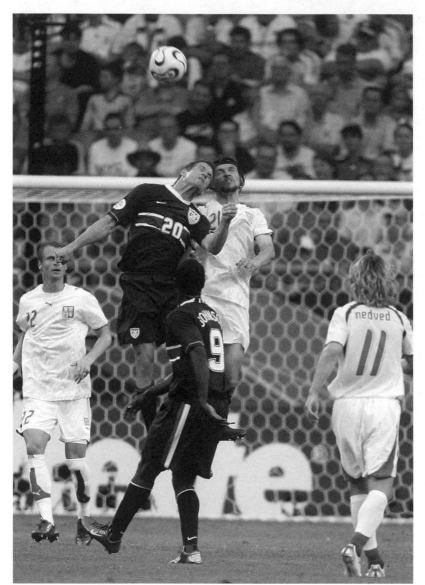

Brian McBride (left) and Tomas Ujfalusi, 2006 FIFA World Cup between the United States and the Czech Republic. Head-to-head contact is one of the most common accidental impacts that can lead to a concussion. (Photograph by Tony Quinn; SoccerStock.com)

cer there are a number of head-to-head injuries; however, in men's soccer there seem to be more elbow-to-head injuries. Players can lose their balance in the air and hit the ground with their head, which can lead to a more serious injury (as in the case of the Algerian soccer player). Thankfully, these more serious injuries are rare in soccer. For high school players, a team might expect a concussion about once every four to five seasons. In college, a team might see upward of one concussion per season. Some high schools, however, report concussion rates similar to those at the college level, and professional teams might see even more. As the level of play increases, so does the incidence of concussion (as with most other injuries). Nevertheless, the incidence of concussion in soccer is lower than in other sports like football, hockey, wrestling, or gymnastics.

Head injuries in soccer are predictable. They usually happen in front of the goal (during a cross or corner kick) where there is congestion of players, or they can happen at midfield during a goal kick, punt, or clear; F-MARC research favors the latter. Of course, head injuries can happen anywhere on the field, but these are the most common locations.

The parent in the stands wants to know, "Can a ball cause a concussion?" Yes it can, from accidental contact. During accidental contact, the neck muscles have not contracted to fix the head to the trunk. Without the neck muscles stabilizing the head, the violent impact of the ball can cause a concussion. These are usually rotational injuries and usually happen when one player mis-kicks a ball, which then strikes the side of another player, or when a player is not paying attention and gets struck by, for example, a punted ball or other such strong kick. Heading is a very complex skill, and at its most important core, the player *must* contract the neck muscles to fix the head to the trunk. If done properly, there is a whole lot more mass overcoming the ball mass. If not, then the ratio of head mass to ball mass can favor the ball.

Field assessment of head injury. Probably the most important thing is to be prepared, and that means know your team. Given the current demographics of the youth soccer player in the United States, there is a good chance that some parent—from either your team or the opposition—is a physician or other healthcare professional. A cell phone or money to make a phone call should be at every game and practice.

I will say this numerous times here. A player does *not* have to be unconscious to have sustained a concussion. Loss of consciousness and memory loss of events surrounding the injury certainly can be indicative of a severe concussion, but other, continuing symptoms may also signal a concussive injury.

When a player gets injured and remains on the ground or staggers and seems dazed, a concussion has probably occurred. Watch closely, as the game may still be going on—the dazed player may get ignored

SYMPTOMS OF A CONCUSSION

Any of these symptoms are an indication of a concussion. These may be evident on the sidelines or in the days afterward. Be aware that some of these symptoms may be "normal" for some players. It is not unusual, for example, for athletes to develop a headache during training or competition. It's not a bad idea to give this list of symptoms to your team and have them fill it out after training. Thus, the player who generally has a headache or feels nauseated after training might need to be queried about other symptoms after sustaining a suspected head injury. In some sideline evaluations of head injury, these symptoms are rated on a 0 (none) to 6 (severe) scale.

- Dizziness
- Headache
- Nausea
- Vomiting

- Balance problems
- Trouble falling asleep
- Sleeping more than usual
- Drowsiness
- Low energy
- Sensitivity to light
- Sensitivity to noise
- More emotional than usual
- Irritability
- Sadness
- Nervousness/anxiety
- Numbness or tingling
- Feeling slowed down
- Feeling like "in a fog"
- Difficulty concentrating
- Feeling "pressure" in the head
- Difficulty remembering things

as play continues. The game may have to be stopped to get the player off the field. If the player stays on the ground, first check the ABCs: check for a clear *Airway*, check for *Breathing*, and evaluate *Cardiovascular* or circulatory status by checking the pulse. If the player is unresponsive, assume there is a neck injury that needs to be stabilized and that the player needs to be transported to an emergency room. *Never move an unconscious player.* Other players may think they are being helpful, but they are the last people you want moving an unconscious player. Players must know to leave an unconscious player to medical personnel.

In sideline evaluation, people commonly ask questions like the date, who is president, and other common knowledge questions. These questions test longer-term memory, not the type of memory typically affected by a concussion. Questions should be about what happened

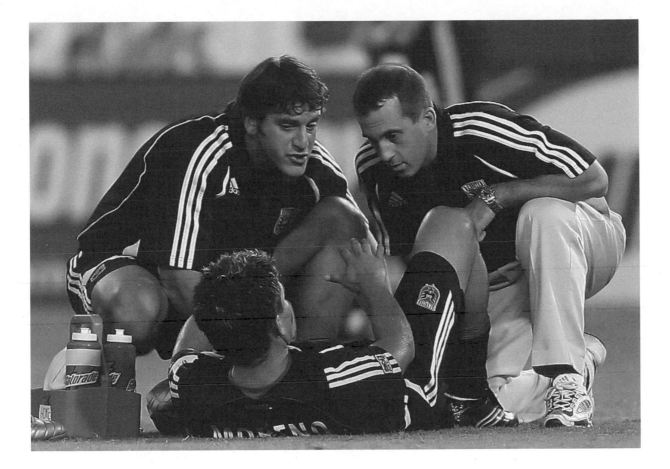

immediately prior to contact: who passed the ball, did you jump, what hit you, who hit you, were you going forward or backward—things like that. Give the player three to five nonsense words to remember. Ask him to repeat them back to you right away. Then ask the injured player to repeat the words again in 5 or 10 minutes, and then again later still. Failure to accurately recall the words is suggestive of concussion. Also, the player must be truthful about symptoms. Any headache, dizziness, or nausea that does not resolve in 15 minutes keeps the player from returning to the game. Always be suspicious because *players will lie to get back into the game*. Have the injured player do some exercise on the sidelines, and ask about symptoms — symptoms are harder to hide with a little exercise (for example, they may shake their head, rub their eyes, or squint). A player with any period of unresponsiveness should be transported to an emergency room. According to U.S. Soccer policy, if the trainer thinks a player has sustained

D.C. United trainers attend to Jaime Moreno in a 2006 match between the D.C. United and the Utah Real Salt Lake. On-field treatment begins verbally. Don't move a player until it is determined that moving him won't make things worse. A referee's desire to keep the game moving is not as important as the player's well-being. (Photograph by Tony Quinn; SoccerStock.com) a concussion, regardless of severity, that player is done for the day. Then the evaluation process begins. This is a very conservative view, but it is the suggestion of such organizations as the International Ice Hockey Federation, FIFA, and the International Olympic Committee.

Some people want to "grade" the severity of injury on the sideline. This is a challenge because there are numerous grading schemes (meaning there is no agreement on the injury within the medical community); some even want to do away with grading scales altogether and instead refer to concussions as "uncomplicated" or "complicated," which raises other concerns.

One player might sustain what might appear to be a minor impact yet have symptoms for days or weeks afterward, while another might be unconscious for a couple of minutes but have all symptoms resolve in a couple of days. On the sideline, who might you have said had the more serious injury? See the problem? Most physicians do not grade a concussion at the time of injury, preferring to wait for a few days to see how things develop.

Nevertheless, some sideline examination is important to detect a concussion because even minor brain injury could sometimes lead to lethal cerebral edema. Moreover, there should always be concern about the more commonplace problem of recurrent head injuries causing prolonged changes in mental performance. *When in doubt, hold them out*, and get injured players examined.

And remember, loss of consciousness is *not* a requirement for a concussion. For an interesting take on concussion, see Chris Nowinski's *Head Games: Football's Concussion Crisis* (2006).

Preventing Concussions

Head protection. Whenever parents of young soccer players gather, the talk can turn to head protection. Indeed, there seems to be a trend toward requiring head protection. One spring season a few years ago, a suburban Milwaukee school district mandated head protection for middle school players, and other school districts and recreational leagues have since followed. There are a number of devices on the market.

There are issues with the *perception* of the problem and the *design* of the products, however. The perception that purposeful heading can lead to brain injury is unsubstantiated. There is no evidence to

GRADING A CONCUSSION

Grading of concussions is open for debate, as demonstrated by the many different grading scales used; some experts are even suggesting that such scales not be used anymore. Here are three scales that are commonly used by sports medicine physicians.

Grade	Cantu	Colorado Medical Society	American Academy of Neurology
1—mild	No LOC, PTA less than 5 minutes	Confusion, No LOC, No amnesia	No LOC, sx less than 15 minutes
2—moderate	LOC less than 5 minutes or PTA greater than 30 minutes	Amnesia, Confusion, No LOC	No LOC, sx greater than 15 minutes
3—severe	LOC greater than 3 minutes or PTA greater than 24 hours	LOC	Any LOC, brief or prolonged

Note: LOC = loss of consciousness; PTA = post-traumatic amnesia; sx = symptoms. Many physicians now don't grade; rather, they describe the injury as "concussion with no PTA, sx, or LOC" or "concussion with PTA, no LOC or sx," and so on.

date that supports that statement. Concussions and repeated heading are two separate entities. Mathematical modeling of heading shows that the ball velocity necessary to cause a concussion in a prepared head (that is, purposeful heading) is far greater than any ball velocity ever recorded (well over 100 miles per hour). [During the Korea/Japan World Cup, I cringed when the color analyst said, as David Beckham was lining up a penalty kick against Argentina, that Beckham could kick a ball 100 miles an hour—100 kilometers per hour (about 60 miles per hour) yes, but not 100 miles per hour.] While no one knows the effects of repeated subconcussive impacts, like purposeful heading, Kevin Guskiewicz at the University of North Carolina has published data showing there were no differences in academic achievement (as SAT scores) or cognitive function tests between soccer players, other collegiate athletes, and control students. The only difference among the subjects was that the soccer players had a greater concussion his-

The Standardized Assessment of Concussion (SAC) can be used to give some objective help in making a return to play decision after a head injury. The best use of this scale is to give it to each player at the start of the season, then one can compare the results to those after a head injury. If players don't do as well as they did in preseason, keep them out. (Modified from M. McCrea et al., *Journal of Head Trauma Rehabilitation*, 1998.)

Orientation (1 point each; 5 points total)
Month
Date
Day of week
Year
Time (within 1 hour)

Immediate memory (player is given five unrelated words; 1 point for each recalled correctly; total of three trials, 15 points total)

	Trial 1	Trial 2	Trial 3
Word 1			
Word 2			
Word 3			
Word 4			
Word 5			

Concentration (4 points total)
 • Reverse digits (State each string in order, 1 second per number. Player repeats the string in reverse order. Go to the next string if the player is correct on first trial. Stop if the player is incorrect on both trials. One point each is given for each string length.)

3-8-2   5-1-8
2-7-9-3   2-1-6-8
5-1-8-6-9   9-4-1-7-5
5-9-7-3-5-1   4-2-8-9-3-7

 • Recite the months of the year in reverse order (1 point for entire sequence correct)

December-November-October-September-August-July-June-May-April-March-February-January

Delayed recall (Approximately 5 minutes after the immediate memory; 1 point each; 5 points total)
Word 1
Word 2
Word 3
Word 4
Word 5

Total score possible = 30 points

The following may be performed between the immediate memory and the delayed recall portions of this assessment, when appropriate:

Neurologic screening
Recollection of the injury
Strength
Sensation
Coordination

Exertional maneuvers
One 40-yard sprint
Five sit-ups
Five push-ups
Five knee bends

tory, yet they demonstrated no problems with academic or cognitive function.

The design of some products is directed at the perception that heading is the issue. These products focus the padding around the forehead of the player, where they would head the ball. When three objects collide (ball, headgear, head), the softest object absorbs the impact—the ball. However, damaging head injuries like concussions come from a hard object hitting anywhere on the head, such as two players competing for the same air ball. Their heads collide, and one or both may be concussed. The point of contact is usually not where the ball would contact the head. The same applies to injuries caused by an elbow hitting the side of the head. One might ask whether padded headgear is sufficient to prevent rotational head injuries when a player is hit on the side of the head. Recent biomechanical research does show that some headgears do reduce the force of a linear impact 20% or more when two heads collide. Furthermore, there are a number of head-to-nose or chin contacts in which a player below jumps up and into the player behind, causing a whiplash type of injury. Head contact with the ground often occurs at the back of the head, when an opponent undercuts the player. Headgear will absorb some of the impact involving two hard objects (such as two heads), especially in a linear collision. No product currently on the market (as of 2006) would protect players from all these injuries. Moreover, simply reducing impact does not necessarily mean fewer concussions.

Within the soccer community the concern is that players wearing head protection might play with more abandon if they think they are "protected." If I had a player who played recklessly because he thought the headgear was protecting him, that player and I would have a serious talk. Anson Dorrance's opinion is that if a player doesn't like to head, wearing headgear won't change her mind, nor will a player who is comfortable heading be more aggressive when heading with headgear. Others may or may not agree. However, it is not unusual for a player with a concussion history to think his headgear is protecting him from another injury.

Future design advancements may improve the protection to the player. There is nothing in Law IV about protective headgear. Law IV simply states, "A player must not use equipment or wear anything which is dangerous to himself or another player (including any kind of jewelry)." FIFA has said that a referee may not use the wording of Law IV as a reason to deny a player using any of the current head protection devices. If the refs let Edgar Davids of the Netherlands wear those goggles, then they will have a hard time denying use of padded head protection.

Rules modification. While the game is universal, and you can step on a field anywhere in the world and play with the same rules, local leagues modify rules to fit their own needs. I know of some local American Youth Soccer Organization leagues in California and elsewhere that have banned heading for under-10 teams. In games with players this young, head-to-ball contact usually occurs in one of three ways: most often off a bounced ball, occasionally from a throw-in, or rarely from an accidental contact (usually a mis-kick). Also, the incidents of actual head-to-ball contact by both teams in a game might (and I stress "might") be counted on two hands at best. So while the league management has the best of intentions, it is banning a skill that is rarely used. As I watch soccer games across the age spectrum, I don't see heading becoming an integral part of the game until middle school. From a coaching standpoint, for players ages five to twelve, there are far more important lessons on which to focus than heading. When I coached under-10, I would give the players exposure to head-ball contact but did not spend time training the skill. How did I expose them? Mostly by having the kids do their sit-ups in pairs and one would softly toss a ball for her partner to head back during the sit-up.

Protect your keeper. The goalkeeper is particularly vulnerable to head injury when trying to take the ball off the foot of approaching attackers. The teammates of the keeper can protect their goalie by running at the same pace as the ball in between the attacker and the ball. Track this ball all the way to the keeper until they know the keeper has the ball. Yes, this is obstruction, but as long as the ball is within playing distance of the defender, there is no foul. If the ball is 5 yards away, then it's a foul, but if the ball is within a leg length, there is no foul. Defenders do this all the time when an attacker is chasing a ball toward the end line. They legally obstruct the attacker to get a goal kick. Do the same thing to protect your keeper.

Common sense. There is one problem with soccer being so universal. Everybody, every age, can play together. Use your common sense:

RETURNING TO PLAY AFTER CONCUSSION

The Concussion in Sports Group has suggested the following guidelines regarding concussion management. I quote their suggestions so there is no doubt about any interpretation (see P. McCrory et al. [Concussion in Sports Group], "Summary and Agreement Statement of the Second International Conference on Concussion in Sport, Prague 2004," *British Journal of Sports Medicine*, 2005):

When a player shows *any* symptoms or signs of a concussion:

1 The player should not be allowed to return to play in the current game or practice.
2 The player should not be left alone; and regular monitoring for deterioration is essential.
3 The player should be medically evaluated after the injury.
4 Return to play must follow a medically supervised stepwise process. A player should never return to play while symptomatic. "When in doubt, sit them out!"

Return to play is a gradual process.

1 No activity, complete rest. Once asymptomatic, proceed to level 2.
2 Light aerobic exercise such as walking or stationary cycling.
3 Sport-specific training—for example, skating in hockey, running in soccer.
4 Noncontact training drills.
5 Full contact training after medical clearance.
6 Game play.

With this stepwise progression, the athlete should proceed to the next level if asymptomatic at the current level. If any symptoms occur after concussion, the patient should drop back to the previous asymptomatic level and try to progress again after 24 hours.

from the Team Doc

THE SIDELINE REALITY OF CONCUSSIONS

Unlike doctors covering major university football or National Football League physicians, most medical personnel attending soccer games do not have a great deal of expertise in evaluating concussions. Earlier in my career, I tended to think that players with a suspected concussion were not taking the mental exam very seriously when in fact some were really unable to respond appropriately. This became more apparent later in the day or week. It may also be apparent in the same game if a player returns to play and performs poorly after a subtle "concussion." It is better to wonder later if a player should not have been withheld from play than to allow someone to play on and later see clear signs of a concussion. And I never heard a player say, "I think I have a mild concussion. You should hold me out."

adults should not be playing with an adult ball with middle school–aged and younger players. The ball and force of contact are too much for the growing player.

And, always, always, always pay attention to the game. Never let your mind wander away from all aspects of the game.

Head Injury and Cognitive Function

There is good data showing that some soccer players do have some problems with concentration, short-term memory, planning, and more. Initially, these deficits were blamed on heading, but a closer look at the studies suggests that there were other reasons for the deficits, such as history of alcohol intake, head injuries, learning disabilities, and playing in the old "leather ball" era when the ball could gain substantial water weight during rainy games. More current research shows that cognitive deficits are related to concussion injury and concussion frequency, not purposeful heading.

The medical community is focusing on what might be called "concussion frequency." Two concussions separated by a year might not be as serious as two concussions separated by only a month. This orientation brings to the forefront the concept of "return to play" guidelines. Remember, when in doubt, hold them out. Schools and clubs should also know the local neurologists with experience in concussions . . . just in case.

Conclusion

In summary, there is no scientific evidence to suggest that heading in soccer is unsafe for adult soccer players. Concussions in soccer are rare and occur from accidental head-to-ball contact or when the head contacts a hard object like the ground, post, head, foot, knee, or elbow. Soccer coaches should always use age-appropriate soccer balls when teaching heading and other soccer skills. In the lab, the current protective headgear designs seem to reduce the impact of contact with a hard surface, but whether this will reduce the incidence of concussion is unknown. Now, if someone wants to see if there are any long-term consequences to heading, look a little bit south. Neck arthritis, reduced range of motion, and bone spurs are far more common in retired soccer players than in the normal population.

Ask most athletes about groin pain, and they immediately talk about a strained (pulled) groin muscle. Groin pain is pretty common in soccer, where up to one in four players has had some type of groin injury in the past (present company included). Pay attention to the sports reports, and you will hear about professional athletes sidelined for weeks with groin injuries that sound a good deal more serious than just a strained muscle. This is a curious injury confined to certain athletes that can keep them out for weeks and lead to surgery and a lengthy recovery.

Players of soccer, ice hockey, tennis, and certain positions in football (e.g., quarterback, defensive back, running back) are among the unlucky targets for this injury. The athlete with this problem will complain of pain during repetitive twisting and turning at a fairly high speed. They rarely can describe a single cause; when I've pulled a groin muscle, I could tell you exactly when it happened. In this so-called sportsman's hernia, what has happened is some tearing and inflammation of tissue very low in the abdomen in the area of the inguinal canal—the traditional location for a hernia in a male.

The doctor will examine for evidence of a hernia with the typical probing through the scrotum toward the abdomen and a thorough series of questions about the pain. The pain is usually described as being of "insidious onset" (meaning it just sort of started to be noticed), in the area of the inguinal canal, may radiate to the testicles or down the thigh, and is aggravated by sharp movements, resisted sit-ups, coughing, or sneezing. The pain may lessen with days or weeks of rest but return when the player resumes training. A traditional hernia shows a visible bulge in the lower abdomen, but the sportsman's hernia shows no bulge, just the complaints of pain. Physicians unfamiliar with the injury will explore many diagnoses, such as osteitis pubis, adductor tendonopathy, stress fracture of the pubic rami, and ilioinguinal or obturator neuropathies. There is no definitive test for the sportsman's hernia (also known as athletic pubalgia and Gilmore's groin), and no X-ray image or other imaging technique will conclusively verify the diagnosis. A herniography (an imaging method to detect a hernia) is not helpful in making a diagnosis and is not used by the knowledgeable physician.

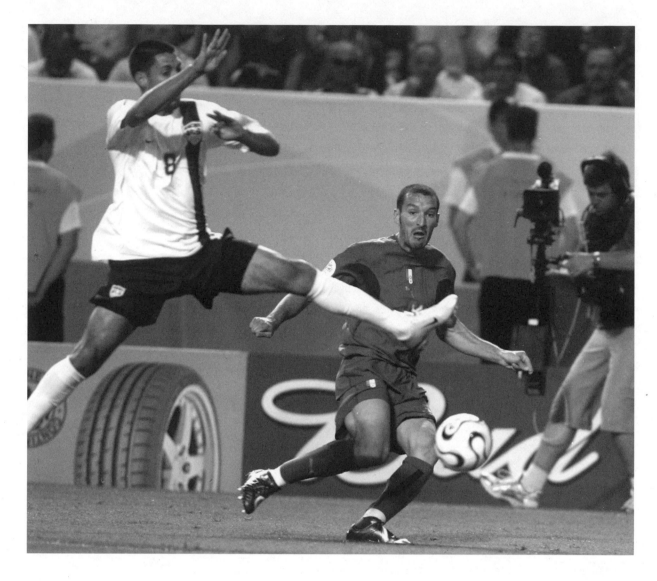

Clint Dempsey (left) and Gianluca Zambrotta, 2006 FIFA World Cup between the United States and Italy. It's no wonder that soccer players need to stretch their groin muscles. (Photograph by Tony Quinn; SoccerStock.com)

So, here is the deal: the player doesn't know how or when the vague pain started, and the doctor is not sure what diagnosis to make, so treatment is a challenge. Conservative methods (rest, stretching, strengthening) are a 50-50 shot at best. Some deep tissue massage techniques have met with limited success. Once all the other possible causes of groin pain have been eliminated, the possibility of surgery might be raised. A routine hernia repair (called a herniorrhaphy) can be performed, though others might do an adductor tenotomy (cutting the tendon of an adductor muscle). These procedures are done by a general surgeon and so far are more frequently performed in Europe than in the United States. General surgeons in the United States are hesitant to do a hernia repair when there is no hernia visible. The reported success rates for the surgery range between 63% and 93%. Patients who were not helped by the surgery often had more than one reason for the pain, so success is linked to a definitive diagnosis. Rehab is a gradual (6–8 weeks) return to ballistic, twisting movements and focuses on improving the strength, flexibility, and stability of the pelvic region.

Three final comments on this injury. First, a sportsman's hernia really needs to be evaluated by a sports physician. Most family medicine physicians and internists will not be familiar with the problem and will struggle with the diagnosis and its treatment. Second, this injury seems to be confined (but not always) to athletes who compete at the very highest levels, mostly professional athletes. Finally, this injury can also occur in women, just not very often.

If this injury is so hard to diagnose and treat, has anyone tried to determine methods of prevention? We look at the literature in the sport where it is most common—ice hockey.

The doctors at the Lenox Hill Hospital in New York City have been studying this injury for a number of years. Before one can prevent injuries, it is important to know how the injury occurs and the general factors of the muscles and joints that differ between injured and uninjured players. On a large group of professional hockey players, researchers measured flexibility and strength of the hip. Then they followed groin injuries over two seasons and went back to their data to see if there were any differences between the injured and uninjured players. This is a common way to study injury prevention.

There was no difference between groups when comparing flexibility, but the injured players had remarkably lower adduction strength (i.e., weaker groin muscles). Does that mean all that time spent stretching the groin is ineffective? I wouldn't go that far. However, it did appear that poor groin strength was a major factor in predicting groin injuries.

The next thing the Lenox Hill folks did was to devise a training program to improve groin strength. (For more information on this program, see T. E. Tyler and S. J. Nicholas, "Stick It to Groin Injuries with Adductor Strengthening," *Biomechanics* 8 [December 2001]: 20–25.) Here is what they came up with:

from the Team Doc
GROIN PAIN

Groin pain is a common complaint among elite male soccer players. For most athletes, acute injuries to the adductor longus or to the rectus abdominis (a pair of parallel muscles that runs from the pubis bone to the sternum) will recover back to normal. Sportsman's hernia, the chronic condition discussed here, is far more difficult to treat. Very strong muscle forces act on the bones around the pubic symphysis (where the two halves of the pelvis connect). The two problems with the symptoms (their insidious onset and the fact that many conditions show the same symptoms) are well recognized but poorly understood, even by many sports medicine personnel.

- *Warm-up*: stationary cycling, groin stretching, sumo squats, side lunges, kneeling pelvic tilts
- *Strengthening*: ball squeezes with different size balls, concentric adduction against gravity (lie on your right side, flex the hip and knee, and plant the left foot on the ground in front of the right leg, then do straight leg raises; don't forget to do the other leg), cable/elastic standing adduction, seated adduction machine, slide board forward, slide board with simultaneous adduction (spread legs and bring both together at the same time), one-legged lunges
- *Ice hockey–specific*: on-ice kneeling adductor pull-togethers (kneel on the ice with the legs spread then pull the legs together), cable crossover pulls, slide skating, cable-resisted striding

Over the next 2 years, 58 players followed the program. Based on pretraining tests, 33 were classified as being "at risk" of a groin injury due to low adductor (groin) strength. The injury rate fell from 3.2 per 1,000 game-exposures (if a team carries 25 players, this would be 3 injuries in 40 games) the two years before to 0.7 per 1,000 game-exposures during the prevention phase. That is a huge reduction in groin injuries.

So what can we take home from this study? Most coaches are pretty good about encouraging flexibility work for the groin, but they need to add some adductor strengthening to team workouts. Players must take some responsibility for strengthening these muscles as well by preparing for the season using some of the exercises listed above. Having had strained groin muscles during my playing days, there is no injury that creates more problems in all aspects of your day. You have no clue how much these muscles are used until you strain a groin muscle. Groin pain keeps players out for weeks while it heals. Wouldn't you rather put in some time preventing this injury rather than spending time on the pine waiting for it to heal?

KNEE INJURIES

After the ankle, the knee is the most injured joint in soccer players. The knee is a delicate combination of simplicity and complexity. It's simple because it's just two bones (plus the kneecap) and two pairs of ligaments, with a pair of cushions in between the bones. It is complex because the joint is far more than just a hinge joint, and it is also the critical joint in the legs when it comes to performance.

The knee's two bones are the femur, or thigh bone, and the tibia, or shin bone. The kneecap (patella) isn't actually connected to either bone but rests in the back of the tendon of the quadriceps muscle. On both sides of the joint is a pair of ligaments, called collaterals (medial and lateral), that prevent the tibia from deviating sideways under the femur. The other pair of ligaments is inside the joint and limits the rotation of the two bones on each other, as well as preventing the tibia from moving too far forward or backward under the femur. The ligaments cross each other, forming an "X," and are called the anterior and posterior cruciate ligaments. The knee's cushions, called the menisci (medial and lateral), sit on the tibia. They are shaped like crescent moons with the open ends facing each other. They help with the stability of the joint and also act as a cushion to absorb the weight of the body above them. The final structural aspect of the knee (and all movable joints) is the articular cartilage that covers the ends of bones that move on each other.

Each sport has its predictable injuries, and not all sports have the same profile of knee injuries. The most common knee injuries in soccer are meniscal tears, ligament sprains (the ACL in particular), and articular cartilage defects.

Meniscal Tears

A meniscus injury can happen by body contact or by twisting or "cutting." The location of pain can help tell if the medial or lateral meniscus have been damaged. Pain with motion, weight-bearing, or twisting movements is pretty common. The diagnosis of meniscus injury is based on pain:

- over the joint line
- over the joint line during hyperextension of the knee
- during hyperflexion of the knee
- during external rotation of the lower leg for medial meniscus injury and during internal rotation of the lower leg for a lateral meniscus tear.

It's pretty common these days for a doctor to order magnetic resonance imaging (MRI). If the diagnosis is uncertain, an MRI can verify

from the Team Doc
MENISCUS INJURIES

Meniscus injuries are common in soccer and can range from occasional localized knee pain to a condition in which it is impossible to straighten the knee without severe pain—a so-called locked knee. Most are treated by excision of the torn portion of the meniscus, which is caught out of place between the femur and tibia, which is what causes the sharp pain and "locking" sensation. Some menisci can be repaired successfully, although many smaller tears occur in portions of the meniscus that do not have a good blood supply and therefore don't have a good ability to heal. Repair is probably most successful in large tears through the peripheral parts of the meniscus, where there is sufficient blood supply and good potential for healing.

the diagnosis, but arthroscopy is the diagnostic and therapeutic tool of choice. Doctors will use an arthroscope to repair or remove damaged cartilage.

from the Team Doc
THE MCL

An injury to the medial collateral ligament makes it very difficult to kick hard with the inside of the foot. Symptoms happen sooner after injury in the game of soccer than in other sports.

Medial Collateral Ligament Sprains

A ligament's job is to prevent a movement, so the best way to damage a ligament is stretch the ligament that is trying to resist a movement to the point of failure. Damage to the medial collateral ligament (MCL) usually happens from a blow to the outside of the knee—the classic "clip" in American football. In soccer the MCL can be sprained during tackles from the side or back when contact is made with the leg and not the ball. The diagnosis is based on localized pain over the ligament and tests of the ligament's ability to resist movement. Years ago, the MCL was surgically repaired, but today, surgery is rare. The player usually follows a rest and slow rehab back to competition, which can take up to 12 weeks.

Anterior Cruciate Ligament Sprains

The ACL gets all the press these days. Most athletes probably think that tearing their ACL is the worst injury that could happen to them. In reality, evaluation, treatment, and rehabilitation of the injury is well hammered out, and many athletes recover completely to make a full return to their prior level of competition. Then again, I know of women who have had four ACL surgeries.

Direct contact to the knee is a minor cause of injury. About 70–75% of ACL injuries involve no direct contact to the knee. The movements are the same motions that players do all the time, like slowing down rapidly, changing direction, and preparing for or landing from a jump. For some reason, the control of the muscles of the hip and knee during these common movements goes haywire. Maybe there was a slight divot in the turf, the player was bumped just prior to the movement, or her concentration was distracted. Something happens to make the planting of the foot different from what was expected. The player may be standing more upright with a straight hip and knee, the thigh muscles contract strongly when the foot is anchored to the ground, the tibia slides forward under the femur, and the ACL tears. It is rare (but not impossible) to tear an ACL on wet ground because of reduced traction, when in a squat (knee bent), or without the foot planted. I've heard of one woman who tore an ACL when she whiffed taking a shot and of a cheerleader who tore the ACLs in both legs when she aggressively extended her knees at the top of a basket toss.

When the ligament tears, there is pain, swelling, and sometimes an audible "pop." Knee stability is poor, and continued play for very long is out of the question. The doctor will do a number of examinations of the knee to confirm that the ACL is torn, and surgery may be suggested. Often the surgery isn't scheduled for about a month after the injury, though the player wants it done *immediately*. Many orthopedic surgeons think the surgery is most successful when it is performed a few weeks after the injury—when the knee is less painful and when walking and motion are more normal. In such cases, there is usually less postoperative pain and fewer problems with rehabilitation. So the player must just sit tight. She is out of play for a while anyway. After a week or two when the swelling goes down, the knee feels pretty good, and she may start wondering whether surgery is still needed. Stay with the original decision.

How is the surgery done? It is complicated, and there are options. A direct repair of the ACL is usually not very successful, so the idea is to insert a tissue (a graft) that is like a ligament (usually a tendon) into the joint where the ACL used to be, to do what the ACL used to do (though this is a huge oversimplification). Most surgeons will drill holes into the femur and tibia at the attachment sites of the normal ACL. The ends of the ACL grafts are then fixed into the two tunnels, and the graft tissue is stretched across the knee into the tunnels to recreate an ACL. Multiple tissues may be used for the ACL graft. The whole procedure takes about 3 hours and is often done in an outpatient setting without an overnight hospital stay.

Articular Cartilage Defects

Articular cartilage protects the ends of bones that move on each other and makes a smooth surface for movement. Under normal conditions, this tissue can last a lifetime, but if damaged it can lead to pain and dysfunction and sometimes to osteoarthritis. Unlike other injuries, the player usually can't recall any specific incident. He just complains of a dull ache in the joint. When a doctor asks about the location of the pain, the player usually just covers the knee with his hand rather than pointing to a specific site, as one might do with a meniscus injury.

In many of the ACL injuries that occur during "contact," player-to-player collisions do not directly damage the knee but instead lead to an awkward or excessive force being generated within the knee as the player lands on the injured knee after being bumped off balance by another player.

The graft tissue used for the ACL varies among surgeons, and surgeons may use different grafts for certain patient groups. Most commonly, grafts come from tissue that is expendable from the knee undergoing surgery. A portion of the patella tendon, with its bony attachment sites from either end, yields a strong graft. Single or double strands of hamstring tendons (semi-tendinosis or gracilis) may be used with a little less pain than with using the patella tendon. The quadriceps tendon from the same knee is sometimes used, as is the patella tendon from the noninjured knee. At times, cadaveric tissue (called an allograft) can be used, but it is not as widely used on younger athletes.

All grafts can be used successfully—and unsuccessfully. There is considerable variability in technique, and an athlete would be well advised to choose a surgeon with a good history of returning athletes to soccer.

The reported success rates for ACL surgery are good, with approximately 85% reporting normal or nearly normal knees. The incidence of re-injury is quite variable. Young female athletes have a higher rate of re-injury than older patients. The previously normal knee is also at increased risk of ACL injury when compared with other athletes with no ACL injury.

The health problems posed by an ACL injury in soccer are considerable. The short-term costs and disability and the longer-term consequences of the injury have prompted much attention toward possible strategies for injury prevention (which will be discussed later).

There is no clear-cut mechanism of injury. Running long distances seems to be a factor. Twisting the knee applies shear forces across the joint, as do quick changes in speed. Soccer players seem particularly at risk due to the running distances and twisting. Basketball and football have the twists but not the running volume. Ice hockey doesn't have the pounding that running requires.

Chondral injuries can affect any articular surface of the knee (femur, tibia, or patella). The lack of cells that can become cartilage and the lack of good blood supply limit the ability of the cartilage to heal. No raw materials equals poor healing.

Symptoms of chondral damage are vague, unlike meniscus injuries, which lead to locking of the joint and a specific location of pain. Often the player will complain of aching knees during or after play. A single traumatic event is rarely recalled. The knee might be stiff in the morning, and there may or may not be any swelling, most common with chronic injuries. Going up stairs is harder than descending

ARTICULAR CARTILAGE INJURIES

Chondral injuries are relatively frequent, especially in high-level soccer players. Often, they present a problem in diagnosis: a meniscus injury may first be suspected, but the MRI fails to show any tear; an injury to the articular cartilage is subtle.

When time and conservative treatment are not resulting in acceptable improvement or function, surgery is often indicated. In many cases, the articular cartilage "peels off" the hard surface of the bone, leaving fragments and flaps that interfere with the smooth gliding function of a joint. The surgical procedures involve a mechanical "cleaning up," or debridement, of the articular cartilage, followed by an attempt to stimulate new cartilage growth. New cartilage stimulation is done most often and most simply by stimulating a bone marrow response by fracturing or abrading through the surface of the newly exposed bone to the deeper vascularized bone. Newer techniques under investigation involve cellular technology—the transplantation of cultured cells of the patient back into the defect.

stairs. Some atrophy of the quadriceps may be present, depending on the length of time the player has had the injury. The ends of the range of motion may be painful. Direct pressure on the kneecap sometimes is painful. No imaging technique is reliably sensitive for detecting this injury, although MRI can be very successful when experienced radiologists use techniques focused on the detection of articular cartilage injury.

The best care usually begins with nonsurgical management. If there is no corresponding meniscus injury, the player usually returns to play, with pain being the main guide. Some players may improve spontaneously, while others may have symptoms for months but are able to continue playing. Nonimpact activities (cycling, swimming) are the best for rehabilitation.

Surgery may be needed to clean up unstable edges or flaps of the torn cartilage. The floor of the defect is usually drilled or scraped to stimulate the growth of the underlying tissue. The tissue that replaces the damaged cartilage is not the same as normal articular cartilage. The defect is usually filled within about 6 months (depending on the size of the defect). Smaller defects that do not affect joint function have a good prognosis. Think of a pothole in the street as a chondral defect on the femur. When a tire (the tibia) rolls over a small pothole, the tire may not touch the underlying pavement, but if the pothole is wide enough, the tire can come into contact with the underlying pavement. Thus, the smaller the "pothole," the smaller the problem with normal knee function; with a larger "pothole," more problems with normal knee function can be expected.

Preventing Knee Injuries

You should see that there are basically two ways to injure a knee—by direct contact to the knee or through noncontact activities. The stronger athlete is better positioned to withstand direct contact to the knee, but in many cases there really isn't a good way to protect a knee from direct contact injury. Of course, with experience, players learn to avoid high-risk situations. (How do you keep from getting your nose broken in two places? Don't go to those two places.) Most of the research is directed toward learning just how a knee sustains a noncontact injury. Once that information is known, methods to prevent the injury can be determined.

Most of this research suggests that landing or cutting is the common action of injury. When a player lands from a jump on a relatively straight knee and hip, the knee is in a poor mechanical position. The knee angle prevents the hamstrings from contracting adequately (which would lessen the strain on the ACL), but the quadriceps can contract very forcefully (which would increase strain on the ACL). If the person is a little off-balance, there may be twisting in the knee that can damage either meniscus. Poor muscle coordination during the landing can lead to the knee buckling inward (knock-kneed landing, or as the Europeans say, X-legged or "kissing knees"), which also places the ACL under added strain and twists the femur in the menisci. If all this happens in just the right sequence, the ACL can tear, and maybe the meniscus can also become damaged.

To see who is at risk, you need to see who lands knock-kneed (X-legged). I have seen this landing when players do a triple standing long jump. From a standing start, the player does a long jump and then on landing does another, then another. Watch from in front or behind. Those who can control their landing will land with their knees over their feet. Those with poor control will land knock-kneed or X-legged. Another method is to have a player drop off a step and land on one leg. Landing with the knee over the foot indicates good control, while a wobbly knee on contact indicates poor control.

There are a number of programs currently under way designed to teach good control. The most visible programs are out of Santa Monica (<www.aclprevent.com>), Cincinnati (<www.sportsmetrics.net>), FIFA (<www.FIFA.com>), Norway, and others. Each uses a series of exercises that can be done during a 10–15 minute training warm-up and has been shown to be very effective. I am not sure that there is anything inherently special about the exercises themselves, just that specific training teaches the player how to control the landing. Today, sports often get players who have had little or no physical education, meaning many players have poor basic motor skills. Many of the exercises are designed to improve basic movement skills.

What type of exercises? Consider the following:

- Zigzag runs, planting and cutting back and forth. Speed is not the issue; control is. Flex the hips and knees, keeping the center of gravity low.
- High knee lift bounding runs where each landing is firm and under control.
- Hopping back and forth across a line on the field. Do these stationary or moving forward and backward. Some people like to make this harder by hopping over a ball, but *landing on the ball can cause injury*, and so I wouldn't suggest using a ball.
- Balance by standing on one leg (make it harder by standing on a folded towel), and toss a ball back and forth.
- Balance by taking a ball through a figure eight around the supporting and free leg.
- Balance by holding the ball, leaning over to touch the ground, and returning to a standing position.
- Stronger hamstrings are important. To strengthen the hamstrings on the field, the player kneels (some would prefer kneeling on a towel), while the partner is behind, anchoring the ankles. The kneeling player slowly leans forward (keeping the back and hips straight) as far as possible (the goal is to get right down to the ground—keep the hands up just in case you need to catch yourself), then

There is no guarantee any training program will make a team injury-free, but there is good information that programs like the F-MARC 11 are very effective. After a general warm-up that breaks a sweat, run through these exercises as a group in about 15 minutes. It may take longer until you and your players learn the routine. (This information, with illustrations, is available online at <http://www.FIFA.com/en/development/medicalsection/0,1236,4,00.html>.)

1 *The bench*

Focus: Core strengthening and stability.

Starting position: Lie on the stomach. Support the upper body on the forearms, and place the feet perpendicular to the ground (like a push-up).

Action: Lift the stomach, hips, and knees so that the body forms a straight line from the shoulders to the heels, parallel to the ground. The elbows should be directly under the shoulders. Tighten the abdominal muscles and buttocks. Lift the right leg a few inches from the ground, and hold this position for 15 seconds. Return to the starting position, and repeat with the left leg. Perform one or two times with each leg. As fitness improves, do more, longer reps.

Important: Do not move the hips upward or let the stomach drop. Keep the body in a straight line.

2 *Sideways bench*

Focus: Core strengthening and stability.

Starting position: Lie on one side. Support the upper body with one arm so that the elbow is vertically under the shoulder and the forearm is on the ground. Bend the bottom knee 90 degrees. When viewed from above, the shoulders, elbow, hips, and both knees form a straight line.

Action: Lift the top leg and hips until the shoulder, hip, and top leg are in a straight line parallel to the ground. Hold for 15 seconds. Return to the starting position, and then do the other side. Perform twice on each side. As fitness improves, do more, longer reps.

Important: Do not drop the hips. Do not tilt the upper shoulder or hips forward. Keep that straight line.

3 *Hamstrings*

Focus: Strengthening the hamstrings.

Starting position: Kneel down with the knees shoulder-width apart, keeping the body straight. Cross the arms in front of the body. A partner pins the ankles to the ground.

Action: Slowly lean forward, keeping the body in a straight line from the thighs to the head. Hold this alignment as straight and as long as possible. When the player can no longer hold the position, use the hands to control the fall. Perform five times. As fitness improves, do more reps.

Important: Do not bend the hips. Perform the exercise slowly.

4 *Cross-country skiing*

Focus: Strengthening the leg muscles.

Starting position: Stand on the right leg, and let the other leg hang relaxed. Bend the hip and knee slightly so that the upper body leans forward. When viewed from the front, the hip, knee, and foot of the supporting leg should be in a straight line.

Action: Flex and extend the knee of the supporting leg, and swing the arms in opposite directions in the same rhythm. Flex the knee as much as possible, but keep the weight balanced on the entire foot. Never lock the knee. Keep the pelvis and upper body stable and facing forward. Perform fifteen times on the right leg, then fifteen times on the left leg. As fitness improves, do more reps.

Important: Keep the pelvis horizontal, and do not let it tilt to one side. Control the knee so that it doesn't buckle inward. Be sure to correct any mistakes in form.

5 *Chest passing in a single-leg stance*

Focus: Coordination and balance; strengthening leg muscles.

Starting position: Two players face each other about 10 feet apart, both standing on their right legs. Knees and hips should be slightly bent. Keep the weight on the ball of the foot with the heel slightly off the ground. When viewed from the front, the hip, knee, and foot should be in a straight line.

Action: Toss a ball back and forth. Standing on the right leg means tossing the ball with the left hand, and vice versa. Catch the ball with both hands, and toss back with one hand. The quicker the exchange of the ball, the more effective the exercise. Perform this ten times on the right leg, then ten times on the left leg. As fitness improves, do more reps.

Important: Always keep the knee slightly bent. Do not let the leg buckle inward. Be sure to correct any mistakes in form.

6 *Forward bend in a single-leg stance*

Focus: Coordination and balance; strengthening leg muscles.

Starting position: Same as exercise 5.

Action: Same as exercise 5. After catching the ball, bend forward and touch the ball to the ground before tossing the ball back to the partner. Perform ten times for the right leg, then ten times for the left leg. As fitness improves, do more reps.

Important: Do not put weight on the ball when it is touched to the ground. When viewed from the front, the hip, knee, and foot of the supporting leg should be in a straight line. Keep the weight on the ball of the supporting foot. Do not let the knee buckle inward. Be sure to correct any mistakes in form.

7 *Figure 8s in a single-leg stance*

Focus: Coordination and balance; strengthening leg muscles.

Starting position: Same as exercise 5.

Action: Before tossing the ball back, swing the ball in a figure 8 around the supporting and free leg. Lean forward when passing the ball around the supporting leg and erect when passing the ball around the free leg. Perform ten times while standing on the right leg and ten times on the left leg. As fitness improves, do more reps.

Important: When viewed from the front, the hip, knee, and foot of the supporting leg should be in a straight line. Always keep the knee slightly bent, and do not let it buckle inward. Be sure to correct any mistakes in form.

8 *Jumps over a line*

Focus: Jumping power and technique.

Starting position: Stand with both feet hip-width apart, about 6–8 inches to the side of a line. Bend the knees and hips slightly so that the upper body leans forward a little. From the front, the hip, knee, and foot of each leg are in a straight line. Arms are slightly bent and close to the body.

Action: Jump with both feet sideways over the line and back as quickly as possible. Land softly on the balls of the feet with slightly bent knees. Jump ten times side to side, then ten times front to back, over the line. As fitness improves, do more reps.

Important: Landings should be soft and quiet. Takeoffs should be quick. Quickness on takeoff and soft landings is more important than jump height. Do not let the knees buckle inward. Correct form is crucial. (My note: I learned this exercise at a coaching school by jumping over a ball, but I have heard of kids landing on the ball and snapping a fibula. Jumping over the line is safer.)

9 *Zigzag shuffle*

Focus: Coordination, agility, and jumping skill.

Starting position: Six cones are set up in a zigzag course, with about 20 yards between each cone. Players start with a shoulder facing the first cone, with the hips and knees bent and the upper body leaning substantially forward.

Action: Shuffle sideways to the first cone, then point the other shoulder at the next cone and shuffle to it, and so on throughout the course. Take off and land on the balls of the feet. Do the course twice. As fitness improves, do more reps on a

longer course (I've seen people modify this exercise by adding carioca reps).

Important: Keep the upper body leaning forward with a straight back. A low center of gravity is important. Land softly and quietly. Do not let the knees buckle inward. Be sure to correct any mistakes in form. Waiting time can be reduced if multiple courses are set up.

10 *Bounding*

Focus: Coordination, jumping power, and technique.

Starting position: Stand on the takeoff leg with the upper body upright. The arm on the same side of the body is forward of the body. When viewed from the front, the hip, knee, and supporting foot should be in a straight line.

Action: Spring as high as possible off the supporting leg. When bounding, bring the knee of the free leg up as high as possible, and bend the opposite arm in front of the body. Land softly and quietly on the ball of the foot with a slightly bent knee. Cover 30 yards twice. As fitness improves, do more, longer reps.

Important: Do not let the knee buckle inward during takeoff or landing. Be sure to correct any mistakes in form.

11 *Fair play*

Important: A substantial number of soccer injuries are caused by foul play, so the observance of the laws of the game and fair play are essentials for the prevention of football injuries.

returns to the upright position. Repeat. Some call these Russian or Nordic curls, and it is a very effective exercise. A child with Osgood-Schlatter's disease might skip this one.

It really isn't hard to dream up other exercises. You need only a few each practice. I find that using this coaching cue is effective: urge the players to run and land quietly. Middle and high school players have especially poor running technique and need constant encouragement to absorb landing forces by bending at the hip and knee. You can't land quietly on a straight hip and knee—you just can't do it.

I am reminded of a story from a presentation on the topic to coaches. The topic was why women basketball players have so many ACL injuries. All the mechanical factors were described and suggestions on training were made. After the talk, this experienced coach (read "old" coach) came up and said basically, "I knew that. Just listen to basketball practice. Women don't squeak their shoes on the court. You can't squeak your shoes standing up straight." We never tell the old-timers anything; they already have the insights. What we can do is quantify what they know from experience.

I'll add one other comment on the topic of prevention. Excellent traction is implicated in ACL injuries. Injury studies that include information about the condition of the surface show that ACL injuries don't occur on wet ground because the traction is so poor (of course, muscle strains rise on a wet surface for the same reason). So while I have no data to back this up, this would suggest doing some training in uncleated running shoes. When players train in uncleated running shoes ("flats"), they run differently because of the reduced traction. They run with shorter strides, chop their steps more when cutting, and lower their center of gravity (bent knees and hips) when turning so that they don't fall. So, do some fitness training and some non-competitive skill training in flats, and then play in cleats (and shin guards) when playing against an opponent. The idea is that the lessons of body control learned from training in flats will carry over to the match played in cleated shoes.

A couple of other general factors about injury prevention in general and knee injuries in particular:

In most U.S. airports I see advertising boards about the increased incidence of anterior cruciate ligament tears in female athletes. The topic can be found in the newspapers, on *SportsCenter*, in *Sports Illustrated*, and more. The following are a few interesting studies:

1 A. Caraffa et al., "Prevention of Anterior Cruciate Ligament Injuries in Soccer: A Prospective Controlled Study of Proprioceptive Training," *Knee Surgery, Sports Traumatology, Arthroscopy* 4, no. 1 (1996): 19–21.

A prospective controlled trial is a good way to study an intervention. Half of 600 male players trained 20 minutes per day, performing increasingly difficult balance exercises. The other half did no supplemental training. The project went for three full seasons. At the end of the study, the trained group had significantly fewer ACL injuries.

Comment: This study is widely referenced as proof that balance training is effective at preventing ACL injuries. Unfortunately, the program didn't work when it was tried in Scandinavia (see study #5 below).

2 David E. Gwinn et al., "The Relative Incidence of Anterior Cruciate Ligament Injury in Men and Women at the United States Naval Academy," *American Journal of Sports Medicine* 28, no. 1 (2000): 98–102.

Sideline discussions about knee injuries in females seem to focus on the fact that there are more women playing, thus the number of injuries should be increasing. The military academies have long served as a research "lab" on a variety of issues because their activities are closely monitored, and all students must participate in physical activity and see the same doctors. In this study, records of ACL injuries at the U.S. Naval Academy were reviewed. The injuries were based on the rates of activity participation for both males and females. In coed soccer, basketball, softball, and volleyball, the female injury rate was 1.4 times that for men. In intercollegiate soccer, basketball, and rugby, the injury rate was nearly 4 times greater for women. In military-specific training, the female injury rate was nearly 10 times that of the male rate. As the intensity of participation increases, the study concludes, so does the rate of ACL injuries in women.

Comment: This is not always the case when staying within a sport. The rates of injury can be pretty high in lower levels of play (at the same age) since the players may not be as physically gifted and may put themselves in risky situations. Nonetheless, the data here are convincing: females tear their knees up at a faster rate than men.

3 John W. Orchard et al., "Rainfall, Evaporation and the Risk of Non-Contact Anterior Cruciate Ligament Injury in the Australian Football League," *Medical Journal of Australia* 5 (April 1999): 304–6.

This little project simply recorded the weather conditions at the time of injury during games (where most injuries occur). Data on 2,280 matches over 6 years were recorded. Noncontact injuries were most common on fields that hadn't had a lot of rain and had rapid evaporation. The conclusion is obvious—a dry field (i.e., one that provides good traction) is a risk for ACL injury. The authors encouraged clubs in areas of low rainfall and rapid evaporation to use extra water on the fields to help reduce ACL injuries.

Comment: Most doctors will say that ACL injuries don't happen in the rain due to the loss of traction. Numerous older and newer studies have shown that athletes who wear the traditional fourteen-studded soccer shoe have a lower incidence of knee injury than those who wear screw-in studded shoes due to the reduced traction of the former. There is no data on the newer bladed shoes on the market today, but I have heard that some professional teams in England prohibit the use of bladed shoes. Traction versus safety is an argument that will continue for some time.

4 Kerstin Söderman et al., "Anterior Cruciate Ligament Injuries in Young Females Playing Soccer at Senior Levels," *Scandinavian Journal of Medicine and Science in Sports* 12, no. 2 (2002): 65–68.

A goal of sports medicine is to prevent injuries. A problem for such studies on active players is the accuracy of reporting. In Sweden, all insurance claims go through one company, Folksam. Population studies on sports injuries severe enough to require an insurance claim are therefore possible in Sweden. The authors pulled records on all female ACL injuries from 1994 to 1998, and then called the players for details about the injury. They were interested in girls who were under 19 years of age. Over one-third of the injured players were under 16. When these younger players were playing with senior players, well over half the injuries were due to contact and were game-related. Over three-quarters had stopped playing soccer 2–7 years after the injury.

Comment: The authors suggested what you have figured out: girls under the age of 16 should not compete in games against senior-level players. Training was acceptable.

5 Kerstin Söderman et al., "Balance Board Training: Prevention of Traumatic Injuries of the Lower Extremities in Female Soccer Players? A Prospective Randomized Intervention Study," *Knee Surgery, Sports Traumatology, Arthroscopy* 8, no. 6 (2000): 356–63.

In this attempt to replicate and improve on the Caraffa study, 121 women were randomly assigned to the control group and 100 to the intervention group (the Caraffa study had no random assignment). The trained group performed similar balance board training as used by the players in Caraffa's study. Nearly 40% of the intervention group dropped out (the Caraffa study made no mention of dropouts—hard to believe there were no dropouts over 3 years). There were no differences in location, type, or severity of injuries between the two groups. The incidence of "major" injuries was greater in the intervention group. In fact, 80% of the ACL injuries in this project were in the intervention group, meaning the balance board training was not successful at preventing ACL injuries. However, players who had an injury in the 3 months prior to the study and were in the intervention group sustained fewer new injuries. Thus, the balance board training was effective at helping the rehabilitation process for recently injured players but was ineffective at preventing ACL injuries.

Comment: This outcome illustrates why studies are done and repeated. This study was performed on women just to see if the original results of Caraffa et al. could be replicated. If one study says something works, it is the obligation of others to try and see if they get the same results. The Caraffa project also had limitations: no random assignment of players to groups and no mention of dropouts. Plus there wasn't any real mention of how exposure was derived.

6 Kerstin Söderman et al., "Risk Factors for Leg Injuries in Female Soccer Players: A Prospective Investigation during One Outdoor Season," *Knee Surgery, Sports Traumatology, Arthroscopy* 9, no. 5 (2001): 313–21.

There are lots of intrinsic factors (anatomy, strength, ligament strength, etc.) and extrinsic factors (field conditions, shoes, traction, etc.) that contribute to knee injury. Nearly 150 women in thirteen teams from two divisions of Swedish soccer were studied for one season. Measurements were made prior to the season, and then factors were reviewed after an injury. The risks for a traumatic leg injury included joint laxity (loose ligaments—a minor factor), postural sway (don't be surprised at how many studies on leg injuries show poor posture is a risk factor), hyperextension of the knees, a strength imbalance between the quads and hamstrings, and a high exposure to soccer (they play a lot). All the players who sustained an ACL injury had a strength imbalance on the injured leg. The strength imbalance was due to weak hamstrings.

Comment: Coaches spend a lot of time on stretching the hamstrings, but nowhere near enough time on strengthening these muscles. Besides, there is also evidence that those with ACL injuries have some of the best ratings of hamstring flexibility.

- Foul play is implicated in nearly a quarter to a half of injuries. Tackles from behind and from the side (when a short pass has been made in traffic) are particularly dangerous.
- Poor flexibility is frequently cited as a risk of injury. Soccer players are notorious for having poor thigh, ankle, and hamstring flexibility, so stretching these areas is important. Nevertheless, players who sustain a noncontact ACL injury almost always have some of the best hamstring flexibility on the team.
- Ask almost any coach who has a few years' experience, and she will tell you that the players with the poorest skills seem to get hurt the most. While most coaches would prefer to coach tactics through small-sided and large group games, there is no substitute for skill improvement. I have heard that some Czech Republic professional teams regularly train with an overinflated (i.e., a "hard") ball for skill training. You have to concentrate on skills to control the ball. When a properly inflated ball is brought out, the ball seems "softer"

and easier to control. I know you all have done this. Play with a regular soccer ball, then play with a volleyball, and you have some pretty good control on the softer ball. Brazilian children often play with a soft, underinflated ball.

- That boy who is at that awkward age in puberty is at a greater risk of injury. During puberty, the boy's height gain occurs at a faster rate than does the muscle mass increase; thus, the boy is tall and "gangly." The prepubertal boy and the boy whose muscle mass has caught up are at less risk of injury. You can't do anything about it—just realize that if you coach in the pubertal years, you will have that gangly boy whose body control is at an odd stage.

- Probably the most important factor in injuries is fitness. Poor fitness is evident when you see that nearly 25% of all injuries happen during the last 10–15 minutes of the game. Study after study that compares injury rates in fit and unfit players shows that the injury rates, serious injury rates, and season-ending injury rates are all smaller in the fittest players. Every player has an obligation to come to training camp in decent condition. They should have followed a program given to them so that they will be most resistant to injury. They should have improved their strength, endurance, and flexibility, along with their skills. Nothing has a bigger influence on injury prevention than fitness.

(LOWER) LEG PAIN: MUCH MORE THAN "SHIN SPLINTS"

Back when I was in high school (way back when), all-weather running surfaces were replacing old cinder tracks. No longer was rain an issue—times were faster, performances improved almost overnight, and we all looked forward to track meets at schools with all-weather surfaces. When one was installed at our school, it wasn't long before some runners were doing their training just inside the track on the grass because they had developed "shin splints." Practically every instance of pain in the lower leg has been blamed on "shin splints," but there are other things that could lead to pain in that area.

During an examination, the doctor considers a "differential diagnosis" or the potential diagnoses that could cause the same signs and symptoms; this is something a doctor does every time he or she examines a patient. There is a lot of anatomy in the leg—muscles, fas-

PREVENTING INJURY

Injury prevention is a neglected part of sports medicine. There is more interest now through the study of injury epidemiology and mechanisms of injury. We do not know enough about injury mechanisms or enough about altering motor performance to avoid injury. We know that knowing how to achieve a very complex motor pattern can improve performance—think of a pitcher's delivery, a tennis serve, or a springboard dive. It appears that we could have some impact on injury prevention if we know simply what to avoid and what to alter.

cia, two bones, blood vessels, nerves, tendons, and ligaments—and all can be the site of some type of pain. So, in no particular order of importance, here are some likely reasons for leg pain. The actual treatments for each are left to the medical doctors.

Stress Fractures

Excessive, repetitive loads can lead to a stress fracture, a very small, but serious, bone injury. Such an injury usually comes about when an abrupt increase in the training load (an increase in frequency, intensity, and/or duration) is coupled with inadequate rest. Rest is when stressed tissues adapt to training; bone adapts by becoming denser and stronger. If rest is too short, the bone can't fully adapt. As muscles fatigue, more of the energy absorbed during impact is transferred away from muscles to the bones. Other factors are implicated in stress fractures like hormonal imbalances, bone diseases, and sleep deprivation. These are more common in women and are part of the so-called Female Athlete Triad (the other two parts of the triad are eating disorders and dysmennorrhea). Routine X-rays only show a healing stress fracture, not a fresh injury. Other imaging studies, such as a bone scan, are better for the diagnosis, and MRIs are also used. The location and injured bone dictate the treatment.

Here are some tidbits about stress fractures:

• Stress fractures are fairly common in soccer players. Nine of twenty-four members of the 1994 U.S. World Cup team had a history of stress fractures.
• The injury was originally called a "march fracture" because it was first noticed in soldiers (in 1855). Stress fractures in sports were first mentioned in 1958.
• The injury is typically seen in inexperienced, unconditioned joggers running fewer than 20 miles a week. They are trying to run too much too soon before their bones have adapted to the new training. If they had started slower and shorter, they might have avoided the injury.
• Women are more likely to develop stress fractures than men, especially in adults.
• The injury incidence is similar between boys and girls under the age of 16.

- Stress fractures account for about 2% of all soccer injuries. Looking at all athletes, the tibia is the most common location for a stress fracture. In soccer players, the most common locations are the metatarsals (second and fifth foot bones mostly), tibia, fibula, femur, and hip.
- Overall, the fractures in the femur and tarsals are more common in older athletes, while those in the tibia and fibula are more common in young athletes.
- Stress fractures seem to be due to training on hard ground, improper shoe selection, training errors, and overtraining.
- Risks of stress fracture include training errors (too rapid an increase in the training dose). Pronated feet or cavus feet have also been implicated. Stress fractures are more common with year-round training. California and Florida have a high incidence of stress fractures.
- In soccer, an increase in the training dose is almost always the culprit. Symptoms gradually increase over 2–3 weeks. Symptoms start out as a dull, gnawing pain, increasing toward the end of a workout. Early on, pain disappears with rest, but as time progresses, pain occurs earlier in the workout and persists well into the recovery period. Pain intensity increases with days of training until running cannot be tolerated. With time, pain will continue into the night. Days off can reduce the pain, but symptoms return with a resumption of training.
- Adequate nutrition is important in treatment. Female athletes may need supplemental calcium. In the female with multiple recurrent stress fractures, an eating disorder needs to be considered. Menstrual patterns need to be determined for possible estrogen treatment. Such treatments should only be undertaken with medical supervision.
- Stress caused the injury, so stress must be removed for healing. It can take 6–8 weeks for the bone to adequately repair itself. Crutches are used if the player has a limp. The player is usually seen in the clinic every 6 weeks during recovery. Once the player is pain-free, he or she can return to training, progressing very slowly.

DEFINING OUR LIMBS

This is one of those definitions that can confuse those who are not in some aspect of medicine. We don't have arms and legs. We have upper and lower extremities. The lower extremity is in two main parts: the thigh (between the hip and knee) and the leg (between the knee and ankle). Ask most nonmedical folks and they will say their lower extremity has a thigh and a "lower" leg. But you already know the proper terminology: when you go to a cafeteria and select chicken, you ask for a thigh or a leg, not a thigh or a lower leg.

from the Team Doc
LEG FRACTURES

There are many ways to treat fractures. Soccer players with displaced fractures (when the fractured ends don't line up with each other) are most often treated with early surgery to stabilize the fracture and to allow some motion. Fractures in the shaft of the tibia (usually due to a kick or a foot-up sliding tackle) often are treated with an intermedullary rod (a metal rod inserted inside the shaft of the bone). Fractures around the ankle are usually due to a twisting injury and are usually stabilized with plates and screws.

Fractures

Tibial and fibular fractures are not all that common in soccer. Most fractures occur in the lower third of the leg. Despite what most people think, shin pads are not designed to prevent fractures any more than a football helmet is designed to prevent concussions. These fractures usually happen from cleats being up during a tackle, especially a sliding tackle, or a really hard blow to the leg. Even though Donovan McNabb fractured his fibula early in a National Football League game a few years ago and still finished the game, when one of these bones breaks, there generally is little doubt.

Shin Splints (or Medial Tibial Stress Syndrome)

Let's go back to 2000 when the women's national team was preparing for the Sydney Olympics. The publicity surrounding the then-reigning world champions constantly mentioned that three starters from the 1999 world championships were recovering from injuries and surgery: Carla Overbeck (Graves' disease), Michelle Akers (shoulder surgery), and Briana Scurry (shin splints). Graves' disease is a treatable affliction of the thyroid (Gail Devers won the 1992 and 1996 100-meter gold medals after having been diagnosed with Graves' disease). Akers dislocated her shoulder after a freak accident while shaking hands with fans during a victory lap. The chance of a youth player being hit with these problems is remote. Scurry's shin splints are another matter. While "shin splints" is a fairly common term, an accurate diagnosis of shin splints is a dilemma. Almost any athlete who has pain in the lower leg will call it "shin splints," but it is not quite that easy.

Pain from this syndrome is usually deep in the leg, down the middle and back of the tibia. Pain comes from some anatomical location, but there is no real consensus on the exact location of shin splints or what actually causes the injury. All the muscles of your leg have some attachment to the tibia or fibula. The common perception is that a change in exercise habits leads to a tearing of the muscles away from the tibia. Some tendon involvement may be present. Bone has a covering called the periosteum (*peri-*: around; *ost-*: bone), and tendon tissue intertwines with the periosteum where the muscle inserts in the bone. Shin splints usually happen to the relatively flat-footed player and may represent increased stresses on the medial tibia or on the muscles preventing pronation of the foot. If the athlete keeps training, the periosteum may pull away from the bone, thus the pain. No one knows for sure if this injury can heal by itself. X-rays are usually normal, and an MRI is still experimental, leaving bone scans as the preferred method of imaging. The actual medical term for shin splints is medial tibial stress syndrome (MTSS) or posterior tibial syndrome.

The typical treatment for shin splints:

- Several weeks of relative rest (do something other than running)
- Nonsteroidal anti-inflammatory medications (e.g., ibuprofen)
- Stretching and thorough warm-up before activity
- Ice massage for 15 minutes after exercise (keep lots of paper cups of water freezing in the freezer)
- Stretching exercises to improve flexibility of the calf and heel cord
- Work on strengthening ankle dorsiflexors (calf muscles)
- Slow, gradual return to running (e.g., progress from water running to Stairmaster to treadmill to over-the-ground running)
- Good-quality running shoes. If an athletic trainer is available, there are some taping techniques that may help. Orthotics may be prescribed. When buying shoes, pick a runner's shop, as the salespeople will be more knowledgeable about shoe characteristics than most salespersons at a "big box" store.

Finally, I've said it before: don't self-treat any pain based on comments in books like these. See a sports medicine physician. Why a sports physician? Unfortunately, there are more serious problems that also cause lower leg pain and can be mistakenly called shin splints, specifically stress fractures and compartment syndromes (which may require surgery). Don't simply shrug off lower leg pain as "shin splints." A sports medicine physician should be consulted.

Chronic Compartment Syndrome

The soft tissues of the leg are contained in four compartments: one in the front, one on the outside, and two in the back. These compartments are enclosed by a very tight tissue, or fascia. The compartment on the front is like a triangle where two sides are the bones and the third side is the fascia. During exercise, the muscles swell with blood, but the fascia and bones restrict how much the muscles can expand. In some people, this fascia is so tight that when the muscles swell

ORTHOTICS FOR SHOES

This condition may improve with custom shoe orthotics. Most soccer shoes do not have much room for an orthotic. This means that a custom orthotic has to be made by a professional who is experienced in fitting these inserts into soccer shoes.

An acute compartment syndrome is a medical emergency and must be treated without delay to prevent tissue death (necrosis). Acute compartment syndromes can happen after direct trauma to the bones or muscles. Chronic compartment syndrome is an overuse problem that does not lead to muscle necrosis.

with blood, they have nowhere to expand, and pain is the result. The diagnosis is made by excluding other causes of pain, as well as by the history of pain; usually the pain increases with exercise and decreases with rest. Should history and physical evidence point toward a compartment syndrome, the doctor may order a pressure test to confirm the diagnosis. A probe is inserted into the muscle on the front of the leg, and a pressure reading is taken at rest and at exercise. If the pressure difference reaches a certain threshold, surgery is suggested.

Other Causes of Pain

Other causes of leg pain include:

- *Proximal tibiofibular instability*: This occurs where the tibia and fibula attach to each other up near the knee—that knot on the outside of your knee about 1–2 inches below the knee. This junction may be disrupted by major trauma.
- *Nerve entrapments*: Any of the major nerves serving the leg and foot can become trapped by muscle contraction or odd arrangements of connective tissue around the nerve. When the nerves become squeezed, it hurts.
- *Tibiofibular synostosis*: A very tight ligament holds the tibia and fibula in parallel. During a traumatic dislocation of the ankle, these two bones could be pried out of parallel enough to damage this ligament. If left to heal on its own, the recovery may lead to a calcification at the point of damage, linking the tibia and fibula by new bone growth. Surgery is required only in cases that do not respond to treatment. You may have heard a variation of this injury, occurring mostly in basketball, called a high ankle sprain by the media.
- *Venous thrombosis*: A thrombosis is a moving blockage in a vein. The pain felt is usually accompanied by swelling in the calf, behind the knee, or in the thigh, and the area may be tender anywhere. You may have heard about baseball pitchers with something like this in their arm; occurrences in the leg are very rare.
- *PVD*: A heart attack is blockage of an artery feeding the heart. Peripheral vascular disease (PVD) is the same thing in the legs. Some forms of exercise can lead to pain that is relieved only by rest. This is a disease of aging not found in the young athlete, but an older relative might mention it when leg pain is discussed.

As you can see, leg pain is a bit more complicated than calling everything "shin splints." To simply call any leg pain "shin splints" may mean someone may be neglecting a problem that is far worse. A physician, in particular a physician familiar with exercise-induced leg pain, should evaluate any circumstances of leg pain.

Overuse Injuries

The main tissue at risk for overuse injury is the tendon. A tendon is the very strong tissue that connects muscles to bones. When it functions normally, tendon is capable of transferring impressive forces from muscle to bone. A tendon is a very dense network of fibers that run parallel to each other along its length. The fibers are bundled, and multiple bundles make up a tendon, which is surrounded by a sheath. In most cases, the sheath, not the tendon, is the problem. The tendon has pretty good blood and nerve supply—not as good as muscle, but better than cartilage.

The diagnosis of "tendinitis" is a bit of a misnomer. There can be some inflammation ("-*itis*") about the sheath, but tendon injuries proper are more correctly called "tendinosis" ("-*osis*" means degeneration). A normal tendon doesn't tear; only a diseased, degenerative tendon tears. There are a number of diagnoses for tendinitis:

Patellar tendinitis
- Patellar tendinitis is commonly called "jumper's knee."
- The pain is usually at the bottom of the patella or in the tendon itself.
- The tendon may feel thicker, and pain often can be reproduced with the athlete lying prone and flexing the knee.
- An extensive rehabilitation program is used to gradually increase stresses on the tendon, including stretching of the quadriceps, hamstrings, and Achilles.
- Muscle strength needs to be increased very gradually, and eccentric work must be introduced very slowly.
- Anti-inflammatory drugs and physical therapy modalities (e.g., ultrasound) may be effective. Therapists have specialized straps and taping that may relieve some symptoms.
- Injections are ineffective. This is a long treatment, and the athlete needs lots of encouragement.

from the Team Doc

A RARE FORM OF LEG PAIN

I've been practicing sports medicine and orthopedics for nearly 30 years. While this synostosis is part of the differential diagnosis of leg pain, I have never seen a soccer player with this condition.

- If treatment is ineffective after 6–12 months, then surgery is sometimes considered.

Quadriceps tendinitis

- Quadriceps tendinitis is less common than patellar tendinitis.
- Rapid acceleration and deceleration can lead to this condition. In younger athletes, a tearing away of a portion of the patella by the quadriceps is more common than tendinitis.
- The tendon is usually quite tender. After a brief rest, the athlete can begin a stretching and running program that does not irritate the tendon.
- Physical therapy modalities and anti-inflammatory drugs are prescribed. Athletes return to play when free of symptoms. Surgery is uncommon.

Hamstring tendinitis

- The constant stopping, starting, and cutting of soccer can also abuse the hamstring muscles.
- Treatment includes activity modification, stretching, strengthening, physical therapy modalities, and anti-inflammatory drugs. In this case, if the inflammation is in a bursa, then steroid injections are helpful.
- 90% of patients usually improve, and the remaining 10% may need surgery.

BACK INJURIES

Injuries to the thorax, back, trunk, abdomen, groin, or pelvis make up about 10% of all soccer injuries. (Many players will complain of back pain, sufficient enough to mention but not severe enough to limit participation. So it's not an injury per se—just a complaint.) The most common back/trunk injury is to the lumbar spine, followed by hip, thoracic spine, and abdomen. These injuries are mostly contusions, mild sprains, or strains. There can be injuries to the internal organs, mostly to the kidneys, spleen, liver, or pancreas, due to player-player or player-goal collision. Blunt injuries are difficult to diagnose and may escape initial detection. Failure to do so can lead to serious complications.

Back pain is very common in soccer players who compete at very high levels. It is most common in players who compete on hard fields; some shock-absorbing insoles might be of assistance. Repeated hyperextension can cause a stress fracture of the pars interarticularis of the vertebral body. The diagnosis is very difficult. X-rays are usually not helpful. Even a bone scan may lead to a false negative diagnosis (the term "false negative" means that the injury is there, but the test procedure failed to find it). A very specialized type of image called a SPECT (single photon emission computed tomography) scan may be needed to confirm the diagnosis. Often a custom brace is needed to prevent hyperextension but may allow an athlete to continue to play.

ANKLE AND FOOT INJURIES

The ankle joint is quite complex, even though most players who sprain an ankle view the injury as little more than a nuisance. The tibia and fibula are parallel bones of the lower leg that form sort of a caliper around the talus bone of the foot, forming the main aspects of the ankle. There are ligaments for stability on the medial side of the joint, from the malleolus (that big bony lump at your ankle). These ligaments are not damaged very often. There are three lateral ligaments (anterior and posterior talofibular ligaments and the calcaneofibular ligament). The most commonly injured ligament is called the ATFL (anterior talofibular ligament; ligament names are a cinch, as ligaments are named for the bones they attach to and their location—anterior/posterior, medial/lateral) on the lateral (outside) side of the joint.

The tibia and fibula are also held together by strong ligaments that attempt to hold the bones parallel to each other. From basketball, we hear about an injury called a "high ankle sprain" that is damage to these tibiofibular ligaments. This injury has serious long-term orthopedic complications if left untreated. So it is wise not to take ankle sprains lightly. Have them evaluated by a physician. The athlete may not be able to tell the difference.

Some comments about ankle injuries from our youth injury study:

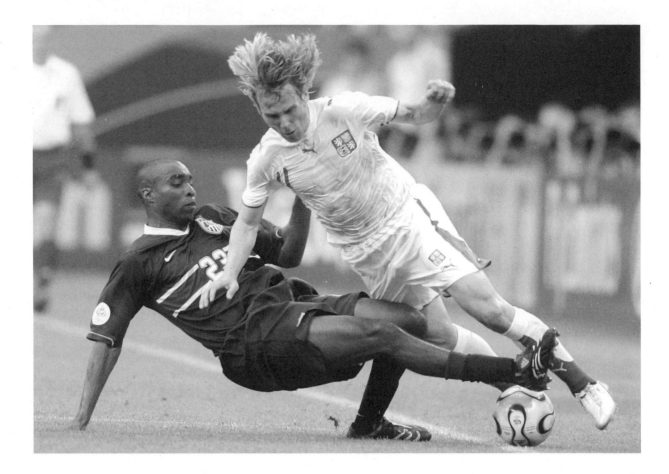

Eddie Pope (left) and Pavel Nedved, 2006 FIFA World Cup between the United States and the Czech Republic. A tackle from the side that comes into contact with the foot or ankle can cause a serious contusion, sprain, or fracture. The pros may do this, but young players need to be taught to challenge from a standing position, not by sliding. Slide challenges are dangerous to both players. (Photograph by Tony Quinn; SoccerStock.com)

- The most common ankle injury was an inversion sprain (where the sole of the foot rolls inward and the outside of the ankle is injured).
- *Over half the injuries were re-injuries.*
- Players injured their ankles due to running/walking—20%, landing—16%, field hazard—11%, being kicked—11%, collision—12%, fouled—6%.
- Players weren't usually changing directions. If they were, the movement was a cut to the side, not a cut requiring the legs to cross over each other.
- When the injury occurred, the player had often lost and then tried to regain his balance (Hmm . . . might taking the fall be the wiser thing to do?).
- Medical research shows that ankle protection absolutely reduces the incidence of ankle sprains in soccer, yet 90% of the injured

INJURIES

players wore no protection. The medical literature is clear on preventing ankle sprains. Supplemental ankle support does little in preventing the first sprain, but extra support is very effective at preventing the next sprain. Braces need to be worn for 6–12 months after the injury, not just a few days or weeks. Yes, ankle braces will stretch out your shoes—a small price to pay to stay healthy.

- Ankle support and proprioceptive training seem warranted. There are a number of ankle supports on the market, and the supports do not affect performance, despite what players say (basketball has a greater agility requirement than soccer, and you see plenty of players wearing supports or high-top shoes). Proprioceptive training teaches the nervous system to control the body and to react to changes faster. Hardly any teams do any training like this. (See the section above on "Preventing Knee Injuries" for examples of such exercises.)
- With over half the injuries being re-injuries, proper and complete rehabilitation is a must to minimize the risk of future injury.

Mechanism of Injury

The ankle is the most commonly injured joint in sports, and most of those ankle injuries involve the lateral ankle ligaments, also called inversion sprains. These happen when the sole of the foot turns too far toward the center of the body. Nearly one in four injuries in soccer are ankle sprains, and wing forwards sustain the most ankle sprains. The ligaments connecting the lateral malleolus to the bones of the foot are damaged when the sole of the foot rolls under the body during activities like cutting or when being tackled. Medial ankle sprains are uncommon but can happen in soccer when a player goes for a tackle, and the opponent applies more force that rolls the sole of the foot outward (eversion). Fractures usually accompany medial ankle sprains. A high ankle sprain is a more exaggerated turning of the foot under the leg, where the talus pries the tibia and fibula out of parallel. In an ankle sprain, the player usually can describe the circumstances of injury pretty accurately. They usually will describe the feeling of a "pop" in their ankle as the talus partially dislocates out from under the tibia and fibula. The joint will be unstable and tender to the touch and will swell rapidly once any restraints (e.g., the shoe) are removed. Ankle fractures can involve any part of either malleoli. A violent external rotation when the foot is in plantar flexion (toes pointed) can break off a piece of a malleolus; imagine an instep to instep hit between two players. Treatment for such a fracture usually involves surgery. Articular cartilage injuries happen in over half of all ankle sprains. Swelling is a common symptom, and sometimes the ankle "pops" during movement.

Treating an Ankle Sprain

Remember, a sprain is an injury to ligaments, and a strain is an injury to muscle, no matter what the color announcer on television says. A sprain means that a ligament has been damaged to some degree, from a small tear to a complete tear through the entire ligament. Thus, treatments are geared toward protecting the damaged ends of the ligament, minimizing edema (swelling), and returning the injured ankle to pre-injury function in terms of strength, range of motion, and neuromuscular control. Between 10% and 20% of ankle sprain injuries lead to residual problems.

Immediately after the injury, the preferred treatment is PRICE — Protect the injury; Rest; Ice; Compression; Elevation.

The ankle is protected by getting the player off the field, and in many cases the player uses crutches on the sidelines. The player is usually asked to sit on the bench for further protection and rest. Ice is applied to the injury to limit swelling and help control pain. Crushed ice is best, and ice water is colder than ice alone. There are many commercial products that can be used in place of ice. The ice is held in place using an "ace" bandage wrapped tightly around the ankle, which adds further compression to the joint. Finally, lessen the effects of gravity (hydrostatic pressure is greatest while standing) by keeping the player seated and the leg elevated, preferably with the ankle above the heart.

One thing to remember about an ankle sprain is that more than the ligaments are damaged. Of importance is the stretch injury to nervous system receptors in and around the joint. This means that the injured joint does not give and receive information as efficiently as it did before the injury. You may have thought that your main senses were limited to pain receptors in the skin, but the information flow to and from the limbs to control the body and execute motor skills is among the most fascinating aspects of skill and sport performance.

With an ankle sprain, the foot and ankle are unable to detect details about the ground, meaning that the player is susceptible to further injury. Never try to just "run it off," as you are at risk for another injury that could be even worse than the sprain. One of the facts we do know from injury surveys is that a minor injury usually precedes a more major injury to that, or another, location.

Rehabilitation

Restoring ankle strength. The muscles that get the most attention are called the peroneal muscles. Two of the three muscles run down the outside of the leg, and the tendons wrap around the lateral malleolus like ropes around a pulley. Look down at the outside of your ankle; tilt the sole of your foot out, and you will see these tendons. There are a number of exercises that a trainer or therapist might suggest. Many of these exercises use elastic bands so you can apply resistance to almost any motion of the ankle. You can hold the elastic, tie the elastic around a chair leg, or loop the band around the foot and work any movement. The therapist might also want work on these muscles through the use of balance activities, like standing on a wobble board (a board with what amounts to half a croquet ball glued to the bottom). After some increase in strength has returned, some functional movements can be added. These frequently involve hopping forward, backward, and diagonally. The therapist will finally recommend some jogging and running before moving into soccer-specific movements with the ball.

I can't say how long it will take to return to play, as everyone is different and the more serious the injury, the longer the rehabilitation. Remember one thing: No matter how stable you think your ankle is, the joint is not back to normal. Most doctors will recommend an ankle support for 6–12 months or more after an ankle sprain. Don't take this piece of advice lightly. Remember, a major injury (and some major injuries can be career-ending injuries) is usually preceded by an incompletely healed minor injury. Who would be willing to risk that just because they don't want to wear some ankle support? Mobility or skill will not be affected by the support. The most widely used braces are the lace-up supports that can be adjusted throughout the game or practice.

Prevention of ankle injuries. There have been a number of studies that look at primary prevention of ankle injuries, and most show no real benefit in preventing a first ankle sprain. Prevention programs (balance boards, neuromuscular training, peroneal strengthening, etc.) are, however, effective at preventing the second ankle sprain. Play the game long enough, and you will probably sprain an ankle, so it is probably okay for everyone to do some ankle-specific training.

A soccer-specific ankle injury. In Europe, an injury peculiar to soccer players is referred to as a "footballer's ankle." Soccer players are known to have ankle instability from repetitive kicking, tackling, pointing the toe to kick hard, pushing off for jumping, and more. The body tries to stabilize the ankle by building up what are known as spurs (little deposits of calcium) that try to limit excess joint motion. Spurs can be found on the talus bone, tibia, or other smaller bones of the upper foot. Players with this diagnosis aren't limited in their sport but may notice it takes a few more steps to "get their ankles moving" in the morning. As the player ages, some loss of range of motion is possible.

Another "Ankle" Injury

A devastating injury to the ankle is an Achilles tendon rupture. This usually doesn't occur before the age of 30. Current data indicate that a normal tendon doesn't tear. Therefore, the ruptured tendon was already degenerating. Treatment for an Achilles tear usually involves surgery. A partial tear is a particularly difficult syndrome to treat. Rehabilitation for either is long and gradual. Certain drugs used to prevent some traveler's gastrointestinal problems (Cipro is the best known of this group of drugs) have been associated with tendon injuries. While I have no data to back up this next statement, I don't know of too many athletes who completely tear an Achilles tendon and return to their previous level of performance.

Foot Injuries

The foot bones are divided into three sets: tarsals (the talus, mentioned above, and the heel, or calcaneus, are both tarsals), metatarsals (the long bones of the feet), and the phalanges (toes). You would think that, given the nature of soccer, foot injuries would be endemic, but foot injuries are not that common. When they do happen, most involve trauma, although a metatarsal stress fracture is an overuse injury. Mature athletes often need a number of steps to work out stiffness and discomfort in their feet in the morning. While this is probably some soft tissue stiffness, morning foot discomfort may just be a factor of age and exercise.

Consider the following foot injuries that most trainers and orthopedists have seen in soccer:

- Midfoot or midtarsal sprains occur along the arch of the foot. This is a rare injury, and the recovery is longer than most anticipate.
- The joint between the tarsals and the second metatarsal (your second toe, this is also called Lisfranc's joint) is the main stabilizer between the tarsals and the metatarsals. Direct trauma (e.g., instep to instep contact) can lead to a variety of fractures or dislocations. The diagnosis is difficult and often missed, meaning treatment is a challenge. Surgery is often required. Don't just assume that pain in the foot is not a big deal. This one can severely hamper development.
- Metatarsal-phalangeal sprains and dislocation happen during repetitive hyperextension of the toes. The athlete notes pain, swelling, and tenderness. PRICE is the treatment of choice. Weight bearing begins when the pain is low enough to be tolerated. Injections to the joint can aggravate the injury and are not used, so be very wary if anyone suggests an injection to the base of your toes. Rehabilitation can be quite long. An orthotic that limits dorsiflexion is sometimes helpful.
- Metatarsal fractures are stress fractures and are not uncommon in the soccer player. Direct forces can fracture the second, third, or fourth (toe) metatarsals. Plantar flexion (pointing the toes down) inversion trauma is the usual cause of fifth metatarsal fractures, especially in basketball players. Metatarsal pads, taping, and a firm boot are used, and weight bearing is as tolerated. Surgery is not out of the question.
- The most common fracture of the foot is a stress fracture. The most frequent locations are the distal tibia or fibula, calcaneus (heel), navicular (a tarsal), and the second and fifth metatarsals.
- Stress fractures are a chronic injury but are noticed because of acute pain. Muscles play a role in shock absorption, and when muscle gets fatigued, the shock absorption patterns shift to more

Stress fractures have for years been the dreaded consequence of playing soccer. It seems that they are less common now, perhaps due to better fields and improved shoe design. Stress fractures are insidious in their onset and don't show up on radiographs (X-rays) for a month or more. An MRI or bone scan is more accurate in the early evaluation of a stress fracture. Most patients are treated with limiting weight bearing, sometimes using a cast or a boot.

The fifth metatarsal is somewhat unusual. The player may describe a history or symptoms in the area. Radiographic studies may actually show evidence of stress reaction in the area of the injury. These fractures often are treated with surgery as the first line of treatment. Some doctors will treat with a cast, and this is also acceptable, but there will be a long period of non–weight bearing.

rigid tissues, like bone. These excessive compressive forces can lead to failure of the adaptive processes of bone during training (yes, bone adapts to training just like muscle adapts). In people with a leg length discrepancy, the shorter leg is most susceptible to injury. Athletes usually complain of a vague pain that comes on gradually.

- Calcaneal stress fractures are very rare, mostly reported in military recruits. If a soccer player complains of heel pain, the most likely cause would be plantar fasciitis.
- Metatarsal stress fractures make up 20% of all stress fractures to the legs. Any of the five metatarsal bones are susceptible. Symptoms progress very slowly, with gradually increasing intensity. It may take 1–2 months before there is any evidence on X-ray. Activity is limited for up to 4 weeks. Water running is helpful to maintain fitness.
- Fifth metatarsal stress fractures require special treatment. 6–8 weeks of non-weight-bearing casting is usually required for a successful return. Surgery is sometimes used to fix the bones, and the athlete may not return for 8–12 weeks.
- Navicular bone stress fractures are a uniquely athletic injury; they just don't seem to happen in nonathletes. The athlete will complain of vague arch pain, pain in the midfoot with motion, and limited ankle motion. All are worse with activity. There is usually tenderness over the navicular bone. If the fracture is not displaced, the treatment is a non-weight-bearing cast. Surgery is required for displaced fractures.
- Metatarsalgia is pain in the metatarsal-phalangeal region of the foot. Frequently it is due to poor foot mechanics from a number of reasons. Orthotics and heel cord stretching are effective treatments.
- We are all familiar with an ingrown toenail, most commonly found on the lateral side of the nail for the great toe. Trauma, poor trimming, and congenital nail growth problems can all be made worse with tight socks or a narrow toe box in the shoes. This can be quite painful and disabling. Why players think wearing a small shoe is helpful is beyond me.
- The slang term for a subungual hematoma is "black nail" or "soccer toe," which is a bleed under the nail from a direct blow. A small

hole in the nail will relieve the pressure and bring almost instant relief. Best let the trainer, therapist, or doctor do this procedure.

A player on your under-12 team develops a cough within the first 5–10 minutes of exercise and has trouble keeping up with his teammates. He might complain of some difficulty breathing and some tightness in the chest, especially when the weather is cold and dry. Smoke, smog, car exhaust, and other air pollutants also make practice worse for the player because you train late in the afternoon when air pollution is at its highest. After practice, things improve, and these symptoms never happen at rest. Mom says she "grew out of childhood asthma" but says her child doesn't have asthma because there has never been any wheezing.

You just might be on the right path thinking the player has asthma, but the perception that wheezing is a necessary symptom is as common as the belief that one has to have been unconscious to have had a concussion (there I go again). Exercise-induced asthma—the more proper term is "exercise-induced bronchospasm" (EIB)—is a fairly common situation. With the number of kids playing sports, it is very likely that coaches are going to have a player with EIB. Therefore, the coach should be familiar with the signs, symptoms, and treatments.

The incidence of EIB in athletes is similar to that of the general population. About 7% of asymptomatic children and around 10% of U.S. Olympians have EIB. The proportions of Olympic medal winners with and without EIB are the same, so EIB is not a limit to performance, if properly treated.

When air is inhaled, it passes through an intricate network of increasingly narrow tubes that carry air deep into the lungs. One class of tubes is called the bronchioles. These have muscle surrounding them, allowing the tubes to narrow or expand depending on the body's needs. In people with EIB, these muscles spasm (thus the term "bronchospasm"), narrowing the bronchioles and trapping air in the lungs. The wheezing of asthmatics comes from their difficulty in exhaling the trapped air.

Certain activities trigger EIB. Higher-intensity exercises with little rest are a problem, like distance running, cycling, basketball, and soccer. Cold weather sports like cross-country skiing, speed skating, and ice hockey also trigger EIB. Activities with longer rest periods, like baseball, golf, tennis, football, and others, are less likely to set off EIB. Swimming is a good activity because the air is usually warm and humid.

A family physician, allergist, or pulmonary (lung) specialist makes the diagnosis. A detailed history of breathing episodes at rest and during activity is critical. To see if the symptoms can be reproduced, the doctor may order some tests, like a controlled exercise test followed by some breathing tests. More definitive tests may be ordered.

The concept of treatment is generally well known: medication that inhibits spasm of the bronchioles. Most drugs are short-acting in the form of an inhalant and can be used in the 10–15 minutes before exercise. They typically last for about 2 hours (such as Proventil, Ventolin, Maxair, Intal, or Tilade). Newer, longer-acting medicines, like Serevent, last up to 6 hours, and Singulair is a pill taken at night. The player with EIB rarely is without his inhaler. Some of these drugs have substances that are banned by various sporting governing bodies, so the athlete that gets to the collegiate or international level will need to notify his medical supervisors.

As in all medical conditions, don't self-diagnose based on a short summary like this. See a physician.

THE FEMALE ATHLETE TRIAD

In the vast majority of sports, men and women compete on a level field. For the most part, both sexes use the same timers, same distances, same rules, and so forth. Thus, coaches of women's teams adopt many of the training procedures used for men. The problem is that while the games and rules are the same, the physiology of each sex is different, and what works for a man might not be as effective for a woman, or worse, the training might actually lead to injuries in women.

Researchers, coaches, and athletes have been concerned about this problem since it became apparent that women athletes sustain far more stress fractures of certain bones (typically tibia and foot bones) than men. If the training was the same, why were women incurring these injuries? The results of these inquiries led to an understanding of the interaction of three factors unique to training women: nutrition, menstruation, and bone health.

The Triad Factors

It is generally assumed that the lighter an athlete, the faster and more efficient he or she will be. In sports where speed or running efficiency is an issue, carrying excess body fat is a liability. Therefore, many female athletes will try to lose body fat to become leaner, faster, and more efficient. The problem is that many female athletes try to lose weight during the time of year with the greatest workload—in season. In addition, to speed up weight loss, they will limit their dietary intake. Both factors are happening at the wrong time of year—in season. As a result, these players end up in a negative calorie balance—they expend more calories (from exercise) than they take in (from food).

A second factor that happens during training in some women is a disruption of the normal menstrual pattern, due to training overloads, caloric deficits, or a host of clinical problems. A word of advice to all female athletes: never assume that menstrual irregularities are due to training. Always consult a physician. When menstrual irregularities happen, the normal cycling of estrogen is upset, and estrogen is an important factor in more than just reproductive health.

The third factor is bone density. Normally, bones become denser (stronger) with weight-bearing exercise (i.e., running). There is another factor that is necessary for improving bone density: estrogen. In the absence of estrogen, bone density decreases to the point where excessive loads (training) actually cause the bone to break down. Normally, such problems don't start happening until menopause, but women athletes with the triad may have the bone density of a woman many years their senior.

The Body's Decision

What appears to be happening is that when a training female athlete limits her caloric intake, the body has to make some "decisions." Does it continue to channel the limited fuel intake to menstrual function or to the muscles for training? If the body chooses the muscles, then reproductive health is pushed into the background, leading to a disruption of normal menstruation and a decline in estrogen levels.

This then leads to a decrease in bone density, with the result being stress fractures. This concept has been referred to as the "energy drain hypothesis."

Avoiding the Triad

So how does one avoid the triad? First and foremost: maintain a healthy diet, and don't try to lose weight in season. Pretty simple, isn't it? Second is to ramp up training slowly. A rapid increase in training is a quick path to injury, especially in athletes who have a low calorie intake and diminished estrogen. Finally, don't try to lose weight during the competitive season.

Is There More to the Triad?

In the triad, the main concern is the effects on bone. The decline in estrogen that comes with irregular or absent menstrual periods leads to a reduction in the density of the bones. The pounding that comes with training can lead to stress fractures—in particular, of the tibia and foot bones.

Yet there might be more repercussions to the triad than just stress fractures. Estrogen is very important to many processes in the body beyond reproductive health. The list of systems influenced by estrogen is quite lengthy: the obvious secondary sex characteristics of females, skin, heart, blood vessels, bone, intestinal function, blood clotting, cholesterol metabolism, the kidney's filtering of sodium and water, uterine muscle mass, and a multitude of other hormones. Guys, don't worry, we are not shortchanged. We produce plenty of estrogen for our needs.

Estrogen has wide-ranging effects. Two different areas of the cardiovascular system may also be affected by a reduction in estrogen and severe calorie restriction: the heart and the blood vessels of the brain.

Heart. Now, this might sound like I am taking things to the extreme. Anorexics have been studied to learn how their bodies adapt to severe caloric restriction. Everyone knows they have lost weight, but much of the weight loss is as muscle mass; it's not all fat mass that has been lost. If the patient loses muscle that controls movement (skeletal muscle), wouldn't it seem possible that other muscle is also lost? The muscle of the heart is very similar to skeletal muscle and also is reduced in the anorexic, pretty much in proportion to the amount of skeletal muscle loss. What appears to happen is that some of the tissue between cardiac muscle cells gets filled with what is called "fibrous tissue," and this fibrous tissue might be at the core of why some anorexics have heart problems. Has this been proven in training females who have been diagnosed with the triad? Not yet. But you have seen some very lean and skinny distance runners. Who is to say that they may not have had some alterations in their heart cells?

Brain circulation. Believe it or not, there is an accepted method to produce a closed head injury in a rat—a very involved procedure. When male and female rats are submitted to this impact, there is a different response. Male rats are far more affected by the impact than female rats. Now, take a group of female rats that have had their ovaries surgically removed (making their hormonal pattern more "male") and perform this standard impact. Guess what? The results of the impact in these female rats are almost the same as the results of the impact in male rats. Reproductive hormones seem to protect the head from injury. The area of the brain that has its function altered is the circulation of blood, meaning the integrity of the blood vessels is influenced by these hormones.

There is very little good data on gender differences in head injuries in soccer players. Some projects show men having more head injuries; others show similar results, and still others report women with more injuries. Much more research needs to be done. But it is not much of a jump to see that a woman who has slipped into the diagnosis of the triad may be placing more than her bones at risk; her heart and brain may also be at risk.

There are dozens of soccer fitness books available.
Here are a few of my favorites.

Arcelli, Enrico. *Nutrition for Soccer Players*. Spring City, Pa.: Reedswain, 1998.

Bangsbo, Jens. *Fitness Training in Soccer: A Scientific Approach*. Spring City, Pa.: Reedswain, 2003.

Csanádi, Árpád. *Soccer*. Boston: Branden, 1967. This coaching book is out of print, but if you find it, you have found the real gem of soccer books. All others pale in comparison.

Dvorák, Jirí, and Donald T. Kirkendall, eds. *International Football Sports Medicine: Caring for the Soccer Athlete Worldwide*. Rosemont, Ill.: American Orthopaedic Society for Sports Medicine, 2005. These are the proceedings of the 2002 FIFA World Cup sports medicine conference.

Gambetta, Vern. *Soccer Speed*. Sarasota, Fla.: Gambetta Sports Training Systems, 1998. There is also a DVD.

Gambetta, Vern, and Gary Winckler. *Sport Specific Speed*. Sarasota, Fla.: Gambetta Sports Training Systems, 2001.

Garrett, William E., Jr., Donald T. Kirkendall, and S. Robert Contiguglia, eds. *The U.S. Soccer Sports Medicine Book*. Baltimore, Md.: Williams and Wilkins, 1996.

Herbst, Dan. *Soccer: How to Play the Game: The Official Playing and Coaching Manual of the United States Soccer Federation*. New York: Universe, 1999.

Ivy, John, and Robert Portman. *Nutrient Timing System: The Revolutionary New System That Adds the Missing Dimension to Sports Nutrition: The Dimension of Time*. North Bergen, N.J.: Basic Health Publications, 2004. This book is about nutrition for strength training.

————. *Performance Zone: Your Nutrition Action Plan for Greater Endurance and Sports Performance*. North Bergen, N.J.: Basic Health Publications, 2004. This book focuses on nutrition for endurance sports.

Kirkendall, Donald T. "Creatine, Carbs, and Fluids: How Important in Soccer?" Gatorade Sports Science Institute Sports Science Exchange #94. Available online at <http://www.gssiweb.com/Article_Detail.aspx?articleid=696&level=7&topic=7> (8 March 2007).

Kirkendall, Don, Sam Snow, Jesse DeMello, and Dave Oliver. *A Guide to Soccer Field Testing*. Lincoln, Neb.: Performance Conditioning, Inc., 2001. Available from the publisher: P.O. Box 6819 Lincoln, NE 68506-0819; (800) 578-4636; <www.performancecondition.com>.

Kleiner, Susan M. *High-Performance Nutrition. The Total Eating Plan to Maximum Your Workout*. New York: J. Wiley, 1996. Susan Kleiner is my favorite sports nutrition author.

————. *Power Eating*. 3d ed. Champaign, Ill.: Human Kinetics, 2007.

Nowinski, Chris. *Head Games: Football's Concussion Crisis*. East Bridgewater, Mass.: Drummond Publishing Group, 2006.

Price, Robert G. *The Ultimate Guide to Weight Training for Sports: Maximize Your Athletic Potential!* Cleveland, Ohio: Price World Enterprises, 2003.

Schum, Tim, ed. *Coaching Soccer*. Indianapolis: Masters Press, 1996. This is a compilation of articles from the National Soccer Coaches Association of America *Soccer Journal*.

Science and Football: Proceedings of the World Congress of Science and Football. London: E. and F. N. Spon, 1988–. These volumes are too expensive for most to purchase. You can find them in a university library. (Call first.)

Verheijen, Raymond. *The Complete Handbook of Conditioning for Soccer*. Spring City, Pa.: Reedswain, 1998.

The following websites contain useful information.

<WWW.FIFA.COM>

Want to kill some serious time? Navigate to the links for the more than 200 member nation websites. Some sites are exemplary, e.g. Belgium. The World Cup 2006 site is terrific for looking at video clips of past competitions; you can see Maradona's "Goal of the Century" at the 1986 World Cup or Pelé as a 17-year-old at the 1958 World Cup in Sweden. Note that FIFA.com is undergoing a major overhaul and is due to launch in June 2007, so some FIFA.com web addresses herein may change. The improved site promises better, easier, and more intuitive navigation.

<WWW.NSCAA.COM>

This is the website of the National Soccer Coaches Association of America, the world's largest soccer coaches' organization.

<WWW.SAYSOCCER.ORG>

This is the website of the Soccer Association for Youth.

<www.soccer.org>

This is the website of the American Youth Soccer Organization.

<www.soccerspecific.com>

This is a membership site for soccer coaches.

<www.TheFA.com>

This is the website for England's Football Association.

<www.ussoccer.com>

This is the website of the U.S. Soccer Federation.

<www.usyouthsoccer.org>

This is the website of the U.S. Youth Soccer Association.

Back injuries, 228, 229

Balance/body awareness, 60–61, 91

Ball going out of play: and change of possession, 7; percentage of game time, 8, 69; and fluid replenishment, 42

Ball in play: percentage of game time, 8, 69; and fluid ingestion, 158

Bangsbo, Jens, 77

Barrieu, Pierre, 82

Beep tests, 132–34, 138

Beer: and postgame fluid replenishment, 44–45. *See also* Alcohol

Blood doping: and red blood cells, 62

Blood lactate level, 98

Blood pressure: and overtraining, 98

Blood tests: for drug analysis, 45

Body fat: and female players, 51–52, 239; measurement of, 52

Body temperature: and function of water, 29, 40; and breakdown of ATP, 64; and warm-up, 80; and heat, 153; and exercise, 153, 154

Body weight: during season, 35, 51; and fluid loss, 40–41, 42, 44, 49, 56, 159; restoring pregame weight, 42; weighing in and out, 42, 44, 160; and creatine, 45–47, 143; and off-season considerations, 51, 105; and female players, 51–52, 239, 240; and ephedrine, 151

Bolowich, Elmar, 84, 180

Bone density, 239, 240

Box-and-one system, 6–7

Brain circulation, 241

Calcium, 52, 223

Capillary density: and aerobic capacity, 78

Carbohydrate replacement drinks, 36–39, 44, 45, 56

Carbohydrates: as energy source, 28, 29; good carbs versus bad carbs, 30; high carbs versus high protein, 30–31; and high-intensity activities, 31; and glycogen replenishment, 33; relationship with stored glycogen, 36; in postgame nutrition, 37, 39–40; quick absorption of, 38; and nutrition of amateur players, 50; and nutrition of young players, 53–54; and recommendations for players, 56; and recovery, 95–96

Carbonated beverages, 39, 45, 160

Carbon monoxide, 165, 166

Carb/protein drinks, 37, 39

Cardiac output, 63

Cardiovascular system: response to training, 63, 123; general improvements in, 75; and anabolic/androgenic steroids, 145, 146; and androstenedione, 150; and particulate matter, 166; and estrogen, 240–41

Carioca, 89, 90

Cereal/pasta: portion size, 36

Cerebral edema, 196

Changes of direction: frequency of, 4; as eccentric exercise, 33; and specificity of exercise, 77; and agility, 91, 130

Cheese/dairy: portion size, 36

Cholesterol, 30, 147, 149

Chondral injuries, 210–12

Chronic compartment syndrome, 225–26

Clothing: sports clothing, 53, 160, 161

Cognitive processes: and speed development, 86–88; and heading, 178, 202. *See also* Mental preparation

Cold-induced diuresis, 162

Cold medicines, 47

Cold stress, 161

Cold towels, 159

Cold weather, 42, 160–62, 238

Competing versus practicing: and development, 16–17

Competition phase, 101

Concentric muscle contraction, 186

Concussion in Sports Group, 201

Concussions: causes of, 177, 191–92, 199, 202; long-term outcomes of, 178; recognition of, 188–89; mechanism of injury, 191–93; rate of, 192–93; field assessment of, 193–96; symptoms of, 194; grading of, 196, 197; prevention of, 196–97, 199–200, 202; Standardized Assessment of Concussion, 198; returning to play after, 201, 202; sideline reality of, 201; frequency of, 202

Conduction: and elimination of heat, 40, 154, 157; in cold weather, 160–61

Continuous Leger test, 132, 133

Contusions, 180

Convection: and elimination of heat, 40, 154, 157; in cold weather, 160–61

Coolmax, 161

Cooperative speed: and speed development, 86

Corruption: and FIFA fair play, 21, 23

Costill, David, 27, 32

Evaporation: and elimination of heat, 40, 154–55, 157; and sports clothing, 161

Exercise: eccentric exercise, 33, 96, 97, 184; fluid loss from, 42; and oxygen delivery, 62–63; and energy production, 66–69; specificity of, 74, 76–77; and body temperature, 153, 154; formula for limits on, 155–56; and metabolic heat production, 161–62

Exercise-induced asthma, 237–38

Eye injuries, 190–91

Fartlek running, 100, 104

Fats: chemical structure of, 28; as energy source, 28–29, 32, 66; good versus bad fat, 30; for lower-intensity activities, 31; portion size, 36

Fédération Internationale de Football Association (FIFA): fair play motto, 21–24; and doping experiences, 139; and creatine, 142, 143; and anabolic/androgenic steroids, 144; and ephedrine, 151; and high altitude matches, 163; and securing of goals, 176; and head injuries, 177, 182; and tackling injuries, 181; and concussions, 196; and head protection, 200

Female athlete triad, 51, 222, 238–41

Female players: and probability of scoring, 12; and running, 51, 59; and nutrition, 51–52, 239, 240; and ACL injuries, 129, 171, 173; and flexibility training, 179. *See also* Women

FEV$_1$ (forced expiratory volume in first second), 164–65

Fibula: fractures of, 180, 224

Field testing: lab testing compared to, 123, 125; for speed, 125–28; for power, 128–29, 135; for local muscle endurance, 129–30; for agility, 130, 138; for anaerobic capacity, 130–31; and strength and flexibility measurement, 173

FIFA. *See* Fédération Internationale de Football Association

Fitness levels: and response to training, 70; and intensity of training, 71–72, 74; and reversibility of training, 77–78; maintenance of, 78–80, 109; and active rest, 100, 101; and year-round training, 105; and injury prevention, 107, 173, 221; training session for, 109–11, 113; rate of improvement in, 113–14; preseason levels, 115–16, 121, 124, 134; and overtraining, 120; club versus college levels, 137

Fitness testing: lab versus field testing, 123–25; reasons for, 124; and endurance, 124, 131–34, 135, 137; field tests, 125–31; resources for, 134; schedule for testing, 134; representative results for, 135; recommendations for fitness testing day, 135, 138

5-10-5 shuttle, 93

5v2: and warm-up, 77

Flat back four defense, 6

Flexibility: requirements of, 61; and reversibility of training, 77; and

muscle strains, 169; and injury prevention, 173, 179, 220

Flexibility training, 119, 173, 179

Fluid-electrolyte replacement drinks, 36, 37, 38, 41, 44, 45, 156

Fluids: function of water, 40; and dehydration, 40, 156; and body weight, 40–41, 42, 44, 49, 56, 159; recommended levels for drinking, 41–42; fluid loss from exercise, 42; guidelines for fluid replenishment, 44–45, 56; and elite players, 48–49; and semiprofessional players, 49; and amateur players, 51; and young players, 53; and referees, 54–55; fluid loss from travel, 55; recommendations for players, 56; intravenous fluids, 156, 157; and heat illness prevention, 158; and cold illness prevention, 162. *See also* Nutrition

F-Marc 11, 110, 188, 214–16

Food and Drug Administration (FDA), 47, 150, 151

Foot injuries, 180, 223, 234–37

Footwork, 13, 91

Formations, 5–6

Forwards: injuries of, 179

Foul play: and injury rate, 173, 175, 179, 220

Fouls: rules for, 3; change of possession by, 7

4-4-2 formation, 6

4v4: as ideal training game, 15; and fitness training, 113; and specificity of training, 117

Free play: shot to goal ratio, 13

Frequency of training: and training

goals, 71; effect on fitness level, 71, 74; and rest, 71, 120; and volume, 72–73; and maintenance of fitness, 78–79; and recovery, 97; as training variable, 108

Fructose, 28, 39

Fruit: portion size, 36

Galactose, 39

Gambetta, Vern, 82, 86, 88–89, 93

Game action speed, 85

General motor skills development: and injury prevention, 171, 213

Genetics: role of practice compared to, 17, 18; and muscle fibers, 69–70

Glucose: chemical structure of, 28; and high-protein diets, 30–31; and high glycemic foods, 38; in high-carbohydrate drinks, 38, 39; and lactate system, 65; and ATPs, 65–66

Glucose syrup, 36

Glycemic index, 37

Glycogen: stored carbohydrates as, 28; depletion of, 31, 32; replenishment of, 32–33, 37, 96; and overtraining, 98. *See also* Muscle glycogen; Stored glycogen

Goalkeepers: and probability of scoring, 12; male and female goalkeepers compared, 13; and training games, 112–13; injuries of, 176, 177, 179; protection of, 200

Graves' disease, 224

Gregg, Lauren, 17

Groin muscles: soreness of, 76; and muscle strains, 185, 203–6

Groin pain, 203, 205

Guaranteed-play guidelines: in youth leagues, 125

Guide to Soccer Field Testing, A (Performance Conditioning, Inc.), 134

Guskiewicz, Kevin, 197

Hamstrings, 185, 213–14

Hamstring tendinitis, 228

HDL (high-density lipoproteins)–cholesterol, 30, 147, 149

Heading: and power, 60; and head injuries, 177, 191, 193, 196–97, 199, 200; and cognitive function, 178, 202

Head injuries: causes of, 175, 177, 179, 180, 182, 188, 193, 199; and head flicks, 175, 189, 190; and heading, 177, 191, 193, 196–97, 199, 200; long-term outcomes of, 178; and cognitive function, 178, 202; vulnerability of head, 188; minor injuries, 189–91; eye injuries, 190–91; and women, 191–92; field assessment of, 193–96; recurrent head injuries, 196; gender differences in, 241. *See also* Concussions

Head protection, 196–97, 199

Heart: and oxygen delivery, 62–63; and estrogen, 240–41

Heart rate: response to training, 63; and intensity of training, 72, 121; and overtraining, 98; and heat, 156; and heatstroke, 157; and cold weather, 162

Heat: and speed of game, 8; elimination of, 40, 154–55, 157; and fluid loss, 42; and young players, 53; and environmental conditions, 153–56

Heat cramps, 156

Heat exhaustion, 40, 156–57

Heat illnesses: prevention of, 40, 158–60; and humidity, 156

Heat injury, 156–58

Heatstroke, 40, 156, 157–58

Heinrichs, April, 13, 133, 134

Hemoglobin: oxygen carried by, 62, 63; and nandrolone, 139–40; and altitude, 163; and carbon monoxide, 165

Hernia, 203–5

High-carbohydrate drinks, 36–39, 44, 45, 56

High glycemic foods: and insulin response, 30; and pregame nutrition, 36; list of, 37; and rise in blood glucose, 38; and postgame nutrition, 39

High-intensity activities: one-third of game in, 5; carbohydrates used for, 31; energy for, 31; and aerobic capacity, 59; and running time, 59, 121; muscle fibers associated with, 69–70; warm-up for, 89; and fitness training, 111; frequency in training schedule, 114–15; percentage of, in training sessions, 116–17; and 4v4 tournaments, 118; and interval training, 119; and player fatigue, 120; and creatine, 142, 143; and ribose, 150; and exercise-induced bronchospasm, 237–38

Hip arthritis, 178

Humidity: and WBGT, 155; and heat injury, 156; and slowing of heat loss, 160; and heat loss in cold weather, 161

Nitrogen oxides, 165–66

Nutrition: role in performance, 27, 33; building blocks of, 27–29, 31; good versus bad in diet, 30–31; match nutrition, 35–40, 48, 49, 56; and vitamins, 42–43; and vegetarian players, 47–48; and traveling, 48, 55; and injury prevention, 48, 105; and elite players, 48–49; and semiprofessional players, 49; and amateur players, 50–51; and female players, 51–52, 239, 240; and young players, 52–54; and referees, 54–55; recommendations for players, 56; off-season considerations, 105; and stress fractures, 223. *See also* Fluids; Supplements

Obstacle avoidance, 91

Offensive formations, 6

Offensive tactics, 7

Off-season training, 94, 103–6, 121, 124, 132, 134

Offsides: rules for, 3

Ohio State University, 161

1-minute push-up, 129–30

1-minute sit-up, 129

Open step, 91

Orthotics, 179, 225, 236

Osgood-Schlatter's disease, 187–88

Osmolarity, 38

Overload: and training, 70–71, 95

Overreaching syndrome, 97

Overtraining syndrome, 97, 98–100, 103, 113, 119, 120, 223

Overuse injuries: and rest days, 71; and recovery, 97; and intensity and duration of training, 113; and

leg pain, 227–28; and metatarsal stress fractures, 234–35

Oxygen: delivery of, 61, 62–63, 67, 123, 150, 163; use of, 61, 63–64, 67, 68–69, 123, 163; and warm-up activities, 81; and altitude, 162, 163; and carbon monoxide, 165

Ozone, 164–65, 166

Pain: and specificity of exercise, 76–77; groin pain, 203, 205; leg pain, 221–28. *See also* Muscle strains

Particulate matter, 165, 166

Passing: role in game, 3, 4; and possession changes, 4, 5; passes per possession, 9–10, 12–13; proportion of completed passes, 13

Patellar tendinitis, 227–28

PC (phosphocreatine), 65, 68

Penalty area: and scoring probabilities, 10, 13; and lateral speed, 91; and head injuries, 175, 182

Perception of exertion: and intensity of training, 72; rating scales, 73; and training, 119–20

Perceptual speed, 85

Performance: and match density, 17; role of nutrition in, 27, 33; and decline in body water and weight, 40–41; and carbohydrate intake, 45; and nutrition of elite players, 48; and physical fitness, 59; and overload training, 70; and cross-training, 75; and overtraining, 98, 120; and training to games ratio, 106; and creatine, 141, 142; and nutritional modification, 151; and dehydration, 159; and altitude, 163, 164; and ozone values, 164

Performance Conditioning, Inc.: *A Guide to Soccer Field Testing*, 134

Periodization: and volume of training, 100, 103, 113; and recovery, 100–101; and planning year-round training, 104; and fitness training, 113; and weight training, 119

Physical fitness: factors important to soccer, 59–61. *See also* Fitness levels; Fitness testing

Pick-up games, 102

Player fatigue: and scoring, 8; and decline of stored glycogen, 31, 32, 48; delay of, through training, 33; and fluid replenishment, 44; and nutrition of elite players, 48; and female players, 51, 52; and overload training, 70; and specificity of training, 74; specificity of fatigue, 75; and overtraining, 98, 119, 120; and sprinting field tests, 127, 128; and muscle strains, 185

Players' abilities: and team playing style, 6

Player-to-player contact: and injuries, 179

Play fair: FIFA fair play motto, 21–24

Play to win: and FIFA fair play, 21

Polylactate: in high-carbohydrate drinks, 39

Portable goals, 176, 177

Portion sizes, 36

Possession changes: and passing, 4, 5; and errors, 7, 8, 15; methods of obtaining possession, 7–8; and small-group tactics, 8; rate per game, 9; and training games, 112; and 4v4 games, 117

Posture: and speed development, 88; and acceleration training, 89–90

Power: requirements of, 60; and reversibility of training, 77; field tests for, 128–29, 135

Practice: and development, 16–17; deliberate practice concept, 17, 18–21, 88. *See also* Soccer practice

Preparatory phase, 100, 104

Preseason conditioning: and injury prevention, 106–7, 173; and English FA, 116, 177

Preseason fitness levels, 115–16, 121, 124, 134

PRICE (protect injury, rest, ice, compression, elevation), 232

Prior injuries, 108, 169

Progressive overload, 70–71

Promoting interests of football: and FIFA fair play, 23

Proprioceptive training, 231

Proteins: as energy source, 29; high carbs versus high protein, 30–31; and ATP, 66

Proximal tibiofibular instability, 226

Punishment: and fitness training, 124

PVD (peripheral vascular disease), 226

Quadriceps tendinitis, 228

Racism: and FIFA fair play, 21, 23

Radiation: and elimination of heat, 40, 154; and heat loss in cold weather, 161

RDA (recommended daily allowance)

guidelines: and food volume, 27; Western diet compared to, 33, 34; athletes' diet compared to, 33, 34, 35, 50–51; carbohydrate/fat/protein percentages in, 33, 34, 51

Reactions: and speed development, 88

Reaction speed, 85

Recognition/reaction, 91

Recovery: and aerobic capacity, 59, 68, 84, 104; between runs, 59, 68–69, 84, 104, 116, 126, 127; principles of, 93, 95–103; and speed training, 94; and overtraining, 97, 98–100; and Yo-Yo intermittent recovery run, 98, 132–33, 134, 135; and periodization, 100–101; and fitness testing, 124, 135, 137; and creatine, 142; and stress fractures, 222, 223. *See also* Active rest; Rest

Red blood cells: oxygen carried by, 62, 63; and nandrolone, 140

Reep, Charles, 4, 9, 12, 13

Referees, 54–55, 175

Reflex: reaction contrasted with, 88

Regenerative training, 97, 109, 120, 121, 123

Rehydration: and fluid-electrolyte replacement drinks, 38; and heat cramps, 156; and heat exhaustion, 157; and heat illness prevention, 159

Repeat 100s, 100–101, 114, 116

Repetition: and speed development, 88, 94

Resistance training: and soreness, 96, 97

Respect: and FIFA fair play, 23

Rest: and frequency of training, 71,

120; balancing training with, 93; and injuries, 95, 106; and overtraining, 99; as off-season consideration, 105–6; and chronic compartment syndrome, 226. *See also* Active rest; Recovery

Restrictions: and fitness training, 110–11, 112, 113; and economical training, 115; and intensity of training, 118

Retraining: slow process of, 78

Reversibility of training, 77–78, 94

Ribose, 150–51

RICE (rest, ice, compression, elevation), 170, 187

Route 1 soccer, 112

Rowing, 118

RPE (rating of perceived exertion), 72, 73

Rules. *See* Laws of game

Running: distance run in game, 3, 4, 5, 51, 59; and stored glycogen, 32, 35, 36; and glycogen replenishment, 33, 96; and high-carbohydrate drinks, 36; and female players, 51, 59; and referees, 54; recovery between runs, 59, 68–69, 84, 104, 116, 126, 127; and aerobic capacity, 59, 84; and high-intensity activities, 59, 121; and energy production systems, 66–67; and cross-training, 75; deep-water running, 75; and specificity of training, 75; technique for, 88–89, 94, 217; and periodization, 100–101; on trails, 102–3; field tests for, 125; and endurance tests, 131–32. *See also* Speed development; Sprinting

U.S. Women's National Program, 134

U.S. Youth Soccer Association (USYSA), 116

Vegetarian players, 47–48

Venous thrombosis, 226

Vertec, 128

Vertical jumps: and power, 60; and fitness testing, 124, 128–29, 135

Violence: and FIFA fair play, 23

Vitamins: role in bodily functions, 29; and well-balanced diet, 42; use of multivitamins, 42–43

Volitional exhaustion, 32

Volume of training: as product of duration and frequency of training, 72–73; and maintaining intensity, 73, 74; and periodization, 100, 103, 113

VO$_2$ max: and aerobic capacity, 59, 78; and lab tests, 124–25; and 12-minute run, 132

Warm-up: and specificity of exercise, 76, 77; general, 80, 81, 83; specific, 80, 81, 83; benefits of, 80–81, 83; and training, 80–83, 121; sample 15-minute warm-up, 82–83; for speed training, 89; for competition, 94; for fitness training, 109; and flexibility training, 119; for fitness testing, 135; and groin muscles, 206; and knee injury prevention, 213

Water: and body temperature control, 29, 40; and high-protein diets, 31; and high-carbohydrate drinks, 36, 38; function of, 40; recommended levels for drinking, 41–42, 44; overloading with water, 42, 160

WBGT (wet bulb globe temperature), 155

WCI (wind chill index), 161

Weather. See Altitude; Cold weather; Environment; Heat; Humidity

Weight training, 97, 105, 119, 142, 143, 144, 149

Western diet: carbohydrate/fat/protein percentages in, 33, 34

Wind speed: and heat loss in cold weather, 161

Women: and total running distance in game, 5, 59; and passes per possession, 9–10; and female athlete triad, 51, 222, 238–41; and posture for acceleration, 89; and ACL injuries, 129, 171, 173, 208–9, 210, 217, 218–20; and creatine, 143; and steroids, 144, 145; and androstenedione, 147, 148; and head flicks, 190; and head injuries, 191–92; and groin strain, 205; female injuries studies, 218–20; and stress fractures, 222, 223, 238–39, 240. See also Female players

Women's Olympic team (1996): training of, 17, 118

Women's United Soccer Association (WUSA), 5

Women's World Cup: 1991, 8; 1999, 6, 8, 12–13, 15, 153; 2003, 153

World Anti-Doping Agency (WADA), 47, 139

World Cup: 1974, 85; 1982, 153; 1986, 8, 153, 162–63; 1994, 151, 153, 222; 1998, 12–13, 15; 2002, 17, 106, 153; 2006, 15, 175, 182

Wrist injuries: of goalkeepers, 176, 177

Young players (under 10 years): and diversity of sports, 18–19, 20; and nutrition, 52–54; and skill levels, 94, 119; and field tests, 125; and heading, 200; and ankle injuries, 229–30

Youth players: and overcompetition, 16, 17, 20–21, 50, 98, 105–6; and multiple teams, 48, 50, 53, 93, 95, 101, 106; injury rate during puberty, 173–74, 221; injuries of, 176–77, 179–80; and tackling, 185; and stress fractures, 222

Youth soccer: role of, 16; schedules of soccer organizations, 20; and postgame nutrition, 39

Yo-Yo intermittent recovery run, 98, 132–33, 134, 135

Zonal marking, 5, 6